16.99

C

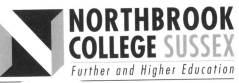

NORTHBROOK
COLLEGE SUSSEX
Further and Higher Education

rmation Services

1903 606213

Outline of Sociology as Applied 606451
ewed,

Outline of Sociology as Applied to Medicine

Fifth Edition

David Armstrong MB BS MSc PhD FFPHM FRCGP
Reader in Sociology as Applied to Medicine, Guy's, King's and
St Thomas' Medical School, King's College London, UK

A member of the Hodder Headline Group
LONDON

First published in Great Britain in 1994 by Butterworth Heinemann

This fifth edition published by Arnold, a member of the Hodder Headline Group,
338 Euston Road, London NW1 3BH

http://www.arnoldpublishers.com

Distributed in the United States of America by
Oxford University Press Inc.,
198 Madison Avenue, New York, NY10016
Oxford is a registered trademark of Oxford University Press

British Library Cataloguing in Publication Data
A catalogue record for this book is available from the British Library

Library of Congress Cataloging-in-Publication Data
A catalog record for this book is available from the Library of Congress

ISBN 0 340 80920 5

1 2 3 4 5 6 7 8 9 10

Commissioning Editor: Georgina Bentliff
Development Editor: Heather Smith
Project Editor: Wendy Rooke
Production Controller: Lindsay Smith
Cover Design: Terry Griffiths

Typeset in 10/13 pt Sabon by Phoenix Photosetting, Chatham, I
Printed and bound in Malta

What do you think about this book? Or any other Arnold title?
Please send your comments to feedback.arnold@hodder.co.uk

C O N T E N T S

PREFACE TO THE FIFTH EDITION

Changes in any academic field arise for a number of reasons. First, new concepts or views of an area emerge that cause old understandings to be refreshed with new insights. In the sociology of health and illness, ideas about the importance of social capital or disablement provide good examples. Second, the gradual accumulation of new evidence in an area leads to a reassessment or a new synthesis. The 'paradox of health' is an interesting example of this: it seems that as people get 'healthier', rather surprisingly, their quality of life may get worse. Third, there are new policies, particularly in the area of health care provision, that require not only describing but also understanding by being placed in a wider context. Clinical governance, managed care and managed competition are policies that about a decade ago were little more than ideas but are now mainstream aspects of health care.

In this fifth edition of the book my aim has been to incorporate these many new developments, which has meant the addition of new sections and editing of old ones. As in the past, the emphasis throughout the book remains on providing a clear framework for understanding the relationship between health, health care and the society in which it occurs.

I remain grateful to the students and colleagues who over the years have influenced the course and form of this book.

David Armstrong
London
2002

chapter 1

INTRODUCTION

At the end of the eighteenth century a new type of medicine swept away the old humoral theories of illness that had dominated clinical practice for hundreds of years. The distinctive feature of the new medicine was its claim that illness existed in the form of localized pathological lesions inside the body (Foucault 1973). It followed that clinical practice could no longer monitor the illness as it entered, moved through, then left the patient's body, but had to devise techniques for interrogating the inner spaces of the body where the disease was located. Thus, the clinical examination was introduced to search for disease, post mortems became common to identify precisely the disease that had caused death, and the hospital emerged as a place for patients to receive treatment.

This new model of disease – often called biomedicine because it reduced illness to a biological abnormality inside the body – led to enormous resources being invested in the examination of anatomical and physiological processes, both normal and abnormal, to identify the underlying basis of pathology. In addition, the pharmacological revolution of the last 50 years has given doctors a wide range of weapons with which to fight these diseases/pathological lesions. Yet despite these many successes, there seem to be some illnesses that have failed to succumb to this biomedical analysis. Many patients report illnesses for which no underlying physical pathology can be found. A good example of this failure is the old problem of insanity or madness: for nearly 200 years, the brain tissues of the mentally disturbed have frequently been examined after death to find the organic roots of their illness, but without success.

Biomedicine continues to hold out hope that eventually psychiatric disorder will be explained in terms of cerebral pathological lesions; but others have argued that the search for a full organic explanation of psychiatric morbidity is futile. No matter how closely the internal electronics of a television set are examined, they will never reveal an adequate understanding of the type and variety of programmes being shown; in the same way, an examination of the brain, no matter how detailed, can never succeed in explaining why someone has a certain thought, or holds a religious or political belief, or speaks a particular language. In other words, there seem to be many aspects of human functioning that fall outside the classical biomedical model. Certainly, there may be neurophysiological patterns coexisting with ideas, thoughts, culture etc., but these biological correlates cannot explain the origins of the content of these mental processes.

Historically, the biomedical model of illness has been extremely successful. Yet in some ways it has been too successful in that it has crowded out alternative explanations and understandings of the nature of illness. There is a limit to how far people can be understood as technical machines and there is now evidence of the vast number of ways in which illness is a problem of the psychosocial world as much as the biological. Even well-defined diseases such as cancer or myocardial infarction have major impacts on patients' social worlds, and medicine needs to attend to these aspects of illness just as much as to the traditional pathological lesion. The arguments in this book attempt to redress the imbalance by identifying deficiencies of the biomedical model and describing various ways that the social world relates to illness.

SCOPE OF THE BOOK

Sociology is concerned with the study of society. This gives it a very broad remit. Everyone is born into a society; that particular society provides, through language and values, the key building blocks of identity; society influences our knowledge, our thoughts and our behaviour. The wide range of 'other' societies and societies in our historical past shows how varied this social context can be.

The wide scope of sociology means that it can contribute to an understanding of medicine in three broad ways.

1　The first is the way that social factors impinge on individuals and groups to influence their health and behaviours. This area is covered in the first part of the book, starting with explanations of how people decide they are ill and need help from medicine and moving into describing the health and patterns of behaviour of social groups. In many ways, discussion of the social factors that impinge on individuals overlaps with health psychology, but, for historical reasons, the study of help-seeking behaviour has been developed by sociologists and it seems a useful place to start, leading in from the familiar figure of the individual to the influence of social group membership.
2　The second is that sociology can stand back from health, disease and medicine and, rather than ask 'how do social factors affect them?', can explore how these concepts themselves are socially established. This approach might be described as the sociology *of* medicine as against the above sociology *in* medicine. For example, different societies have different 'systems' of health care, different views of what constitutes health and different ways of thinking about the nature of illness. This approach is best illustrated in the final chapter, though it informs ideas in several others such as the chapter on the health care professions and models of illness.
3　Finally, sociology has something to say about the way health care is provided and evaluated. In part, this analysis overlaps with economics, social policy and epidemiology but, notwithstanding the dangers of encroachment into the territory of other disciplines, this book offers chapters on how health care is organized and how it can be evaluated.

Chapter 2

GOING TO THE DOCTOR

The traditional medical model holds that disease is a lesion inside the human body that produces two types of indicator of its presence:

1 *symptoms*: those feeling states patients experience that alert them to the possibility that all is not well (e.g. pain),
2 *signs*: those pointers the doctor identifies that signify the existence of the underlying pathological lesion (e.g. tenderness).

The doctor is therefore a sort of detective who infers the existence of the disease from the outward clues of its presence. The patient is required to report the symptom to the doctor so that the detective work can proceed. Unfortunately for the efficient working of this model, people do not behave according to expectations in that they do not seem to use symptoms as triggers to seek help. This pattern of behaviour shows itself in two ways.

1 There are people who fail to go the doctor, or go very late despite experiencing symptoms of serious disease. This group constitutes what has been termed the 'symptom iceberg', in that it seems that there are more people who have serious symptomatic disease not under medical care than there are receiving treatment (Hannay 1979).
2 There are people who attend the doctor with relatively minor or trivial complaints. Some general practitioners (GPs) have reported that between a third and a half of their patients fall into this category (Cartwright and Anderson 1981).

So the 'obvious' view that when people feel ill (i.e. experience symptoms) they are inclined to visit the doctor looks mistaken, or at least only forms part of the picture. Symptoms are not, therefore, simple cues for action.

THE EXPERIENCE OF SYMPTOMS

A novel survey, published in 1954, described the views on health of some 500 families in a small American town (Koos 1954). The study reported that people seemed to experience symptoms much more frequently than their rate of medical consultations would indicate. The researchers were surprised at this finding because they had assumed, as had medicine for a century and a half, that symptoms as indicators of disease almost invariably led to help-seeking behaviour.

In the following years, other researchers made similar discoveries. Sometimes patients were shown a checklist of symptoms and asked whether they had experienced any of these: for example, one such survey found that adults could recall on average about four symptoms in the previous 2 weeks (Dunnell and Cartwright 1972). Other surveys simply asked whether any symptoms had been experienced in a certain time period, making the assumption that, as it was patients who made the decision whether or not to view a symptom as serious, they were best able to judge what was to count as a symptom in the first place. Also, some researchers persuaded people to keep a daily 'health diary' of the symptoms they experienced; many found that noting down at least one symptom every day was not uncommon (Banks et al. 1975).

Table 2.1 shows the results of one study of patients' reported symptoms and their decision to consult a doctor. It can be seen that the decision to seek medical advice was a relatively rare occurrence, even for supposedly serious symptoms such as chest pain.

Table 2.1 Ratio of symptom episodes to consultations

Headache	184:1
Backache	52:1
Emotional problem	46:1
Abdominal pain	28:1
Sore throat	18:1
Pain in chest	14:1

After Banks et al. (1975).

From these surveys of symptom prevalence, a number of conclusions can be drawn:

- symptoms are very common,
- reporting of symptoms is related to how they are measured,
- most symptoms are not taken to the doctor (if they were, the health service would be overwhelmed),
- something more than a symptom/feeling ill is necessary before people will visit a doctor.

So why *do* people go to the doctor?

ILLNESS BEHAVIOUR

In 1960, the notion of 'illness behaviour' was advanced to explain the process by which patients came to seek medical help or advice (Mechanic and Volkart 1960). Illness behaviour was a term describing:

the ways in which given symptoms may be differentially perceived, evaluated and acted upon (or not acted upon) by different kinds of persons   (Mechanic 1962).

For Mechanic, the task was to persuade patients to behave with the same rationality as medicine, to bring serious illness to medical attention and ignore or self-treat minor and self-limiting illness. As he explained: 'one of the prime functions of public health programmes is to teach populations to accept and behave in accordance with the definitions made by the medical profession'. But this was quite unrealistic. Patients had not been through medical school, so how could they know which symptoms signified serious disease? And besides, this was to assume that medical definitions were always the right ones for every patient.

However, first the factors affecting the 'career' of moving from being a well person to being an ill patient had to be better understood. The 'symptom iceberg' had shown that, as symptoms were so widely distributed, they could not be the precise trigger that took people to the doctor (Hannay 1979); nor did it seem to be the symptom's severity or seriousness, as the 'clinical iceberg' contained patients with serious diseases (Last 1963), and their accompanying symptoms, who chose not to go to the doctor.

Following Mechanic's original work, various studies explored the factors that encouraged or hindered people's attendance at medical facilities. Each of these studies contributed to understanding the question of why patients choose to see their doctor. As ever, in understanding human behaviour there is not one simple explanation but rather a range of ways of looking at the problem.

A DECISION-MAKING MODEL

A decision-making model sees patients as rational decision makers who weigh up alternatives before deciding whether to visit the doctor. This process involves two strategies: first there is an evaluation of the symptoms, then there is a consideration of possible alternative courses of action.

Are my symptoms normal or abnormal?

Symptoms and their perceived danger are subjected to some form of evaluation. Because frequent background symptoms are a normal event for most people, it tends to be the symptom that is unusual or atypical in form or context that is seen as most threatening.

- Certain symptoms are classified as normal probably because of their wide prevalence in society. Headaches, for example, are so common that only about 1 in 200 is presented to the doctor; those that turn up are presumably unusual in some way, perhaps in terms of frequency or context.
- Normality may not only be defined by reference to the total society, but also to smaller groupings within the community. Everyone belongs to a number of social subgroups and will therefore tend to accept the expectations of these groups with regard to symptoms and illness. For example, one of the expectations of old age is that more general aches and pains will be experienced than

in younger people. The experience of such symptoms may be seen as normal by many old people and many may be tolerated without bothering the doctor. Even when the patient presents to the doctor, this 'normalization' may block the emergence of important diagnostic information. While taking a medical history from a patient who smokes, it is not uncommon to find the existence of a cough is denied. On prompting, he (and, increasingly, she) often remonstrates, 'Oh, its only a smoker's cough'. The patient has interpreted 'Do you have a cough?' as 'Do you have an abnormal cough?'.

- Earlier events may also be called upon to normalize the presence of a symptom. For example, a rodent ulcer might be seen as a bruise that has not healed from an earlier bump on the forehead, or the lump of a breast cancer might be explained away by some half-forgotten injury; as it grows very slowly in size, its characteristics are not seen as abnormal as it 'has always been like that'. It is occasionally only when the cancer breaks down and fungates that the patient comes to the doctor complaining of the unacceptable smell.

What else can I do?

There is a variety of alternative strategies (that are not mutually exclusive) available for people who experience symptoms. Some of these are covered in more detail in Chapter 10.

- The patient may ignore the symptoms.
- The patient may consult with friends and relatives. Advice given by friends and relatives constitutes a *lay referral system*, analogous to the medical system, in which the patient is referred to lay consultants with successively greater claims to knowledge or experience of the symptom in question. A study of the use of lay networks in primary care found that 70 per cent of patients consulted with friends and family before their consultation with the GP; on average, patients consulted with 3.6 other people (Cornford and Cornford 1999). No doubt such networks limit the demand for medical services, as most symptoms are probably self-limiting.
- The patient may use self-medication or self-help.
- The patient may consult with professional health care practitioners.

Whether the last course of action is pursued and formal health care approached can be seen as a process by which the patient compares the relative costs and benefits of such action.

What are the costs and benefits of seeing the doctor?

The first decision concerns the perceived value of going to the doctor: will he or she be able to do anything for the problem? Patients will have their own idea of what treatment the doctor can offer and this will in its turn influence the decision to consult. Some people consult their doctor expecting cures and treatments that do not exist; alternatively, many people do not consult because they feel the doctor cannot do anything for them. One study investigated the experiences of a group of patients in the last year of their lives, as reported by their family, friends and carers. Many symptoms had been experienced for which no medical advice was sought: 29 per cent of these symptoms were described as 'very distressing' and 37 per cent had been present for a year or more (Cartwright 1973).

In many countries, a visit to the doctor incurs financial cost and no doubt this is a disincentive to seeking medical advice. However, even when there are no direct financial penalties, there may still be significant other costs that might deter the patient.

- Opportunity costs: what else could the patient do, considering the time and travel costs incurred in seeing the doctor?
- Inconvenience costs: waiting times and waiting lists, inconvenient clinic times, uncomfortable waiting areas, noisy environments, negotiating past the receptionist etc. might all weigh heavily for the patient, especially if the health problem seems to be relatively minor.
- Interpersonal costs: is seeing the doctor a positive experience? Or is it more of an ordeal? Undoubtedly, many patients are put off going to doctors because they believe they will not get sympathy for their complaint. It has been found, for example, that many patients withhold serious complaints from their doctor because of his or her apparent busyness or disinterest.

SECONDARY GAIN

Obtaining treatment, empathy or reassurance might be high on a patient's list of possible benefits, but in addition a more indirect benefit is the label of being ill. This can be expressed in terms of the 'secondary gain' of visiting the doctor. Just as in mediaeval society people with problems might seek asylum in the cathedral, so in modern society being 'ill' confers a status that might give a patient refuge from life's difficulties.

Being ill can bring advantages for the patient, in terms, say, of sympathy or being excused from some task or responsibility. However, by and large, these benefits only follow from having an illness identified by a doctor. This means that visiting the doctor can result in secondary gain through being labelled as ill. In other words, only the doctor (in Westernized societies) has the social authority to legitimate illness and admit the person to what Parsons described as 'the sick role' (Parsons 1951; see also Chapter 15). According to Parsons, in accepting the sick role the patient gains two benefits but is expected to fulfil two obligations.

The patient is temporarily excused his or her normal role

Being excused from some task or responsibility is the main secondary gain of visiting the doctor. This may be formally recognized by the issuing of a sickness absence certificate. More informally, just being able to say that it was necessary to visit the doctor confers legitimacy on a claim to be sick. Whereas 'feeling unwell' might be treated sceptically by friends and colleagues, a visit to the doctor may be sufficient to gain credibility.

The patient is not responsible for his or her illness

A second benefit of going to see the doctor is that patients are generally not held to be responsible for their illnesses (though see below). Whereas for other life problems such as difficulties in employment, finances or relationships people tend to be viewed as at least partly responsible, illness does not carry this burden. So, if a patient is faced by the misery of a financial problem, who better to offer non-judgemental support for the accompanying depression than the doctor?

The patient must want to get well

By gaining two advantages from the sick role, the patient must meet two obligations. The first is the recognition that the sick role is a temporary status that the patient must want to leave behind. If the patient apparently does not want to get well, then instead of the sick role being conferred by the doctor, a label of 'malingering' may be used.

The patient must co-operate with technically competent help

The fact that it is only the doctor who can legitimately confer the sick role ensures that 'technically competent help' tends to be confined to the formal medical services. A patient who chooses to defer to a lay person with claims to medical knowledge, in preference to a medical practitioner, is judged as not fulfilling one of the basic obligations of the sick role.

While undoubtedly the notion of the sick role is very useful in understanding the behaviour of many people who consult their doctor, its use is circumscribed by those patients who for various reasons are unable to fulfil all the expectations and obligations that it entails. This has been noted as particularly pertinent for patients with a chronic illness who are both unable and unlikely to meet several of the obligations – although this failure to encompass patients with chronic illness may explain why doctors often view chronic illness as less medically interesting than acute illness (reflected in their preferences for the 'acute' specialties, such as general medicine and surgery, against those dealing with chronic problems, such as care of the elderly).

Also, ironically, as medicine attempts to offer more health promotion and illness prevention advice, it begins to undermine one of the key benefits of the sick role. A patient who has been advised to give up smoking but declines and then gets lung cancer might be held to be responsible for his or her illness. Equally, a patient who gets human immunodeficiency virus (HIV) through unsafe sex might be seen as undeserving of the sick role.

SOCIAL TRIGGERS

It is not symptoms themselves that take people to the doctor but the assessment of them. It is possible to break this assessment down into what Zola described as five 'social triggers' that together encompass the various ways in which symptoms come to be seen as abnormal (Zola 1973).

- Perceived interference with vocational or physical activity. As vocational or physical activity is a part of 'normal' life, symptoms that interfere with it must be abnormal. Allowance needs to be made for the type of work or activity: a cut finger may interfere more with keyboard work than with driving a car, and a physical disability may only become apparent to a sedentary office worker if he plays a game of football one day.

- Perceived interference with social or personal relations. Similarly, symptoms that interfere with normal social interaction will be more likely to cause concern. Again, the person's social routines and lifestyle will determine which symptoms are disruptive.

- The occurrence of an interpersonal crisis. An interpersonal crisis can upset the everyday equilibrium many people seem to have with their symptoms. Some change in personal relationships can alter the perception of an otherwise minor symptom or seemingly decrease the tolerance to chronic pain or disability. The patient with long-standing osteoarthritis who presents with joint pain after 'coping' for a long period may, for example, be triggered by a domestic crisis rather than by an exacerbation of the underlying condition.

- A kind of temporalizing of symptomatology. Irrespective of whether the symptom interferes with work or social relations, it may still be seen as unusual or ambiguous. Some deadline may then be set for the symptom. This may be a time deadline such as 'If this symptom has not disappeared by Monday, I shall go to the doctor', or it may be a frequency deadline such as 'If I have more than two nose bleeds this week . . .'.

- Sanctioning. Sanctioning refers to pressure from friends or relatives to visit the doctor. It is not uncommon for a patient to open the consultation with, 'I did not want to bother you but . . . insisted I should come'.

IMPORTANCE OF ILLNESS BEHAVIOUR FOR THE DOCTOR

The answer to the question 'Why do people go to the doctor?' is not a simple one. Studies in the field of illness behaviour have shown that seeking medical help is not necessarily related to the occurrence or severity of a symptom. The way in which a symptom is 'processed', both in individual and social terms, will determine what action is finally taken. Of course, not all patients follow the same pattern or take the same factors into consideration. Their decision may not even seem rational to doctors, but then they may not be aware of the often complex reasoning that brings a patient to the consultation. The patient who seems offhand, the patient who says he or she did not want to come but was sent, the patient who hands over a piece of notepaper with a list of symptoms are all to be understood in the context of a decision-making process that has often gone on for several days or weeks before the patient actually reaches the doctor. To establish during the interview why the patient has come at that particular time may be of great value in both understanding and managing the presenting problem.

Perhaps the patient has unrealistic expectations of the doctor's ability and shows unusual tolerance of different symptoms. A patient may have failed to keep an appointment because the surgery was too far away, because the receptionist was too brusque or because the doctor did not offer the expected sympathy last time. The social trigger may give some clue as to the other reasons why a patient has consulted besides the presenting complaint.

While the doctor always enquires of the particular presenting problem so as to infer the nature of the underlying pathological lesion, it is also always possible to make a 'second diagnosis': why did the patient come *now*? Patients very rarely come to the doctor immediately a symptom starts; most delay and wait hours, days or weeks, even months or years. For example, patients with the chest pain of a heart attack delay an average of 10 hours before seeking medical advice, and even those with a past history of ischaemic heart disease, who should be more aware of the significance of chest pain, act no quicker (Rawles and Haites 1988); no doubt many never seek help at all. In many cases, the actual process of becoming ill that has been described above may be more important in understanding and managing the patient's problems than the illness itself.

This means that on many occasions it is not the illness that the doctor must treat but the social trigger or reason for secondary gain. In effect, in some situations the patient may be using the symptom to gain access so that other problems can be discussed. In this scenario, the symptom is not particularly important and is simply being used as a 'ticket of entry'. Clearly, it is important that the doctor identifies the cues and focuses on the right problem.

ILLNESS BEHAVIOUR AND THE MEDICAL MODEL

Studies of illness behaviour have been very useful in understanding the decision-making processes surrounding the patient's experience of symptoms, and the idea of a second diagnosis has often helped solve an apparently confusing problem. However, the assumption behind most studies of illness behaviour is that patients react in some way to given symptoms. This view that symptoms are somehow 'given' has been challenged in three areas by:

1 psychophysiological studies,
2 interpretive studies,
3 anthropological studies.

PSYCHOPHYSIOLOGICAL STUDIES

Medicine has always linked symptoms to underlying pathophysiological processes, and ultimately to diseases. For example, tiredness suggests anaemia, or low thyroxine, or chronic infection. Pain might arise from inflammation, or from ischaemia. Yet, although a symptom might seem to be the outward manifestation of an underlying pathology, on closer examination the relationship is not so clear.

- Patients can experience a wide variety of symptoms without any apparent underlying lesion: for example, in many instances of angina the coronary arteries seem normal; in half the cases of appendicitis the appendix is not inflamed;

in most cases of backache no structural lesion can be found; tiredness seems more associated with low mood than with anaemia – and so on. Of course, it can be argued that in many of these cases it is just a matter of time before the true underlying lesion is identified, but nevertheless the range and extent of these anomalies are very wide, and certainly it would appear that many cannot be explained by the logic of the traditional biomedical model.

- There have been laboratory studies of the effect of physiological change on symptom perception that suggest there is a rather poor correlation between the two. People seem to be very poor discriminators of their underlying physiological state (Pennebaker 1984).
- Psychological studies of the experience of pain suggest that the connection between tissue damage and pain is not necessarily linear. In his classic study of pain in wounded soldiers, Beecher found that the circumstances surrounding the pain – for example whether they would be returning home or not – was an important factor in the amount of pain that was experienced (Beecher 1959). Similarly, Egbert showed that post-operative pain could be reduced simply by explaining the surgical procedures to the patient before the operation (Egbert et al. 1964).

These various studies of pain lend weight to the 'gate control theory' that claims that the experience of pain, irrespective of the state of stimulation of peripheral nerve endings, is mediated by 'central' brain processing (Melzack and Wall 1965). In other words, the psychological and social state of the individual has a major influence on the pain experienced.

Taken together, these various studies and observations, clinical, physiological and psychological, suggest that symptoms should not be regarded as sort of 'pop-up' indicators of physical abnormality. Symptoms are percepts; they are interpretations by the mind of what is going on in the body. Certainly some of these percepts are closely linked to bodily malfunction – there is probably evolutionary logic to that – but equally many percepts would seem to have little direct relationship with what is actually going on inside the body.

This view of symptoms challenges many traditional medical assumptions. Symptoms are not simply present or not present; they may even become present if the person is asked to think about them. Moreover, people cannot be said to 'interpret symptoms', because symptoms are already interpretations (otherwise it is a case of interpreting interpretations!). Believing oneself to be ill or in need of medical advice would appear to be a more complex process than either biomedicine or the model of illness behaviour described above might suggest.

INTERPRETIVE STUDIES

A core assumption of illness behaviour, like medicine before it, was that symptoms were 'given': patients had symptoms or they did not. It was possible to use questionnaires, checklists and diaries to record the existence of symptoms and calculate their number and type, but of course asking questions in this way always produced a predicted response. Such questions either incorporated the researcher's meanings or pushed the respondent's own views into an inappropriate box. Thus people could be persuaded to provide an answer to the question 'How many symptoms did you experience last week?' or 'Have you had a headache in the last fortnight?', but how valid was the response?

The challenge to this mechanistic view of symptoms came from those who argued for the importance of the meaning that patients ascribed to bodily events. It was the meaning placed on an experience that caused it to be labelled as a symptom and possibly fed back into the experience to make it better or worse.

A formal questionnaire with pre-configured answers – like a multiple choice examination paper – was not the way to reveal these meanings. The new approaches to exploring the experience of illness relied on in-depth interviews to establish the psychosocial context that surrounded the emergence of symptoms into consciousness. These studies found that patients carried out complex exploration and negotiation of experience and meanings, which the acceptance of symptoms as 'given' had failed to illuminate (Locker 1981). Patients seemed to be using their own idiosyncratic personal constructs to evaluate and interpret bodily feelings. Equally, patients' non-compliance (or non-adherence) with recommended treatments might appear as irrational behaviour for medicine, but becomes a rational action from the patient's point of view (Donovan and Blake 1992).

ANTHROPOLOGICAL STUDIES

When medical anthropologists investigated illness in non-industrialized societies, they found that people tended to use complex models to explain their maladies. These explanatory models seemed to offer answers to such questions as 'Why me?', 'What caused the illness?', 'Why did it begin at this particular time?', 'What will be the outcome of this illness?' and 'What should be done about it?'. It was then realized that these sorts of questions were asked by *all* patients, including those in Western industrialized societies. The answers that different patients provide for these questions are known as lay theories of illness or patients' explanatory models.

The origin of individual lay theories is probably threefold:

1 *idiosyncratic*, based on the patient's own observations and experiences;
2 *popular*, derived from the 'lay health system': the social network (or lay referral system, see above) itself sustains various belief systems and explanatory models of illness;
3 *expert* models of illness, in the main from biomedicine, which have an influence on lay theories, but obviously those aspects of expert knowledge that are integrated into a lay context may still appear incoherent to the experts themselves; indeed, experts may have their own lay theories that might be quite opposed to the theories they advance while in the role of expert.

Lay theories have been investigated in a variety of diseases. The range of these studies can be shown by citing some findings.

- One study found that a sample of less well-educated working-class mothers tended to report a fatalistic view of the aetiology of illness. These views would have particular relevance for health education programmes that are based on the notion of disease prevention (Pill and Stott 1982). For example, why give up smoking to reduce the risk of cancer if you believe that whether you get cancer or not is already predetermined in some way?
- Another study of beliefs about the causes of cancer found that a group of patients with cancer had stronger beliefs that cancer had little to do with personal behaviour (many thought it was inherited) than a matched group of patients without cancer. The authors suggested that this particular belief was probably a means of defending against self-blame as a mechanism of coping with a terminal illness (Linn et al. 1982).
- An investigation of what patients with high blood pressure thought the term 'hypertension' meant found that many believed it was caused by too much 'tension' or stress in their lives. Despite the lack of scientific supporting evidence, it was also found that even the experts' model (of the doctors) was sympathetic to the role of stress as an aetiological agent (Blumhagen 1980).
- Finally, a study of lay beliefs about upper respiratory tract infection (URTI), particularly as the basis of the aphorism 'feed a cold, starve a fever', found that such illnesses were analysed in terms of hot–cold and wet–dry to establish the supposed origin of the illness, the meaning of its symptoms and the most appropriate remedies. For example, a cold might be caught by going out with wet hair or from sitting in a draught. Compared with the rather limited medical account of URTIs (chance contact with a virus), these lay explanatory models offered more sophisticated explanations and greater help in deciding how to manage the problem (Helman 1978).

Lay theories are often difficult to pin down because they vary so much between people and within the same person over time. Nevertheless, they are important because they affect health behaviour and doctor–patient interaction. The patient does not come to the doctor with the odd isolated symptom but with a comprehensive belief system that in its range and power rivals the biomedical scientific belief system of the doctor. Therefore, although on the surface the doctor–patient relationship might be characterized by common interests and a common goal, it can be seen to represent a meeting of two different 'experts', each with their own explanations about the nature of illness, its causes, its prognosis and its appropriate treatments (Tuckett et al. 1985).

These new insights into the nature of symptoms and illness have many implications for medicine. At the community level, patients seem to have a 'lay epidemiology' through which they are able to explain the distribution of illness in a population and the specific risks carried by individuals (Davison et al. 1991). Notions such as luck, fate and destiny, though unrecognized by medicine, seem to play a large part in lay people's views of illness – and consequently their likelihood of availing themselves of conventional health promotion messages.

At the individual level, the exact role of symptoms in signifying disease – even when they are taken to the doctor – is much less clear than the biomedical model would suppose (see Chapter 9). However, in terms of the traditional illness behaviour that exhorted the doctor to make a second diagnosis of 'Why has this patient come now?', it is possible to add another question: 'What are the patient's explanatory models which brought about this visit and what implications do they have for the management of the problem?' (Kleinman et al. 1978). Medicine has its own questions about causes, diagnoses and appropriate treatments, but patients have, in addition, another set of questions that might be summarized as 'Why me?', 'Why this (illness)?' and 'Why now?'. These patient questions surely deserve as much recognition as the medical ones.

Chapter 3

MEASURING HEALTH AND ILLNESS

Research in the field of illness behaviour has shown that patients make their own personal assessments of their health status in the process of deciding whether to seek health care. This patient view is not necessarily the same as the medical view of health: it is possible for a patient to feel healthy and a doctor to think otherwise, and vice versa. In effect, doctor and patient might be said to be assessing different components of health: one the biomedical basis, the other its more subjective aspect.

This difference of perspective between doctor and patient reflects the fact that health has many dimensions. This can be a problem when trying to measure health status for purposes of research (Is drug X better than drug Y?), evaluation (Does this service improve patient health?), or resource allocation/needs assessment (Which group of patients is most in need of health care?). Ideally, any definition or measurement of health needs to take account of these different components. In practice, there is no single measure of health that embraces them all, but rather a variety of different ones, each with its own strengths and weaknesses.

MORTALITY

CRUDE DEATH RATES

With the registration of all deaths in the mid-nineteenth century, it became possible to establish the mortality experience of the whole population. At first it was simply a question of adding together all deaths to produce an overall figure, so enabling the mortality in one year or one geographical area to be compared with the mortality in another.

The problem with these mortality figures was that the population 'at risk' of dying varied from year to year and between different areas; the mortality figure therefore needed to be expressed as a rate per number at risk. To achieve this, the raw number of deaths was divided by the denominator of the population's size. This produced what is called the crude mortality rate.

AGE/SEX-CORRECTED MORTALITY RATES

The crude mortality rate is one measure of illness in a community that allows populations of differing sizes to be compared, yet it ignores the fact that the age and sex make-up may be very different. For example, many countries have geographical areas that are popular with elderly and retired people, and these areas, as might be expected, tend to have high crude mortality rates. It is possible, however, that after allowing for this age and sex difference, the actual mortality is not significantly higher than in another part of the country. In consequence, demographers have standardized the death rate by allowing for the age and sex mix of the underlying population. Thus, a crude death rate is adjusted to the rate that would have pertained had the population had the same age/sex mix of a reference (usually the national) population. This statistic is commonly expressed as the Standardized Mortality Ratio, in which the observed death rate is divided by the expected rate based on that population's age/sex mix then multiplied by 100.

AGE-SPECIFIC AND CAUSE-SPECIFIC MORTALITY RATES

Analysis of a population's mortality can be taken a step further with a closer look at age-specific death rates and causes of death. A commonly quoted age-specific death rate is the infant mortality rate (deaths of children under 1 year old multiplied by 1000 and divided by the total number of live births during the year), which is frequently used to assess improvements in the health of a population over time and to compare the health status of different countries. Similarly, because the cause of death is recorded on all death certificates, it is possible to produce death rates for any cause. Again, these can be used to compare the types of illness that kill people both over time and between geographical areas.

Mortality rates have some major advantages as measures of health:

- They are routinely available, by age, sex, cause and geographical area.
- The overall figures tend to be very reliable, given that death is an unambiguous state and all deaths get recorded.

However, they also have serious disadvantages.

- The assignment of a cause to each death seems to change with developments in knowledge and fashion. Thus, to some extent, the differences in the cause of death over time and between geographical areas may be the consequence of different reporting procedures from clinicians, pathologists and coroners.
- They do not indicate the amount of *morbidity* (i.e. illness) in the population. In principle at least, it is possible for a population to have relatively low mortality rates yet include large numbers of people with chronic illnesses, such as osteoarthritis, that do not themselves cause death but are seriously debilitating.

Nevertheless, given the ease of measuring and obtaining mortality data, they are sometimes used as crude proxy-measures of illness, particularly when deciding whether one geographical area has a greater 'need' than another for additional health care resources (see Chapter 12).

MORBIDITY PREVALENCE STUDIES

As medicine has traditionally defined illness in terms of pathology-based diseases, measuring pathology directly would seem to be as good a way as any of assessing the health of a population. This does not mean counting the illnesses in a hospital or clinic, as this would provide a biased estimate (see 'Caseload' below). Ill people outside hospitals have also to be included – hence the idea of community prevalence surveys in which the health status of random samples of the population is assessed. In practice, such surveys pose several difficulties.

* They tend to be very expensive: large numbers of health personnel are needed to carry them out.
* There can be difficulties in defining exactly what is to count as the disease for the purposes of the study.
* It is difficult to allow for severity: two patients may have the same disease but be differently incapacitated by it.
* There is a problem of data comparability, in that it is difficult to add and compare different diagnoses. For example, if one population has 100 cases of ischaemic heart disease and another 100 cases of chronic bronchitis, which is the healthier?

These limitations mean that large-scale community prevalence studies to measure the health of a population are uncommon and, when they do occur, tend to focus on individual diseases that have easy and specific diagnostic tests (such as diabetes).

The major exception to this general rule is psychiatric disorder. The diagnosis of mental illness does not require a technical diagnostic test but relies on the patient's response to the psychiatrist's questions. This has led psychiatrists to try to reproduce the diagnostic interview in a questionnaire. There are now many such questionnaires in existence, perhaps one of the best known being the General Health Questionnaire that is used to identify cases of anxiety and depression in community studies (Wright and Perini 1987; Bebbington et al. 1997).

SICKNESS ABSENCE RATES

A good measure of health status would reduce all illness to a simple figure that could then be standardized by using a common denominator: the health status of one population could then be compared with another. Sickness absence promises such a statistic in that it reduces illness to a number of days lost from work through illness. This latter figure, divided by the number of days worked to establish a rate, can then be used to compare two or more populations or one population over time.

While sickness absence rates are regularly collected and can be obtained for specific geographical areas or time periods, there are problems with their validity:

- They are known to be affected by illness behaviour: it seems likely that some people – and there may be a systematic pattern – are more likely than others to seek work absence for an illness.
- The requirements for sickness certification change over time and vary for different occupations, therefore changing the need to register.
- Perhaps most importantly of all, sickness absence figures only cover that proportion of the population in the workforce. In other words, they exclude children, the unemployed, the elderly and housewives, who, ironically, are believed to have more illnesses in comparison with the rest of the population. In effect, sickness absence rates measure the amount of sickness in the healthiest group in the population.

For these reasons, sickness absence is judged to be a very limited measure of health status.

CASELOAD

One method of measuring illness would be to count the number of times patients in a population visit their general practitioner or attend hospital. Such data could be obtained relatively easily from hospital and general practice statistics. However, these caseload data reflect three different phenomena.

1 They obviously indicate health status, which is what the health measure is trying to cover.
2 They also reflect illness behaviour: it is now well established that many patients with serious illness choose not to seek help from health services, while many with so-called trivial illnesses attend regularly. Explanations for this are discussed in the preceding chapter.
3 The core assumption underlining the use of caseload as a measure of illness is that patients who are ill will seek help for their problem. This depends on patients responding to their illnesses, but it also assumes that the health services are available to meet the patient's need. In practice, access to health services can vary considerably across geographical areas and for different types of illness. Accordingly, the numbers of people being treated partly reflect the need for such treatment, but also its availability: if there are no such treatments available, then, according to caseload figures, there would appear to be no need!

It is almost impossible to disentangle the above three phenomena. Low caseload figures may reflect a healthy population, or they may reflect a shortage of health care to cope with an ill population. This means that, in general, caseload cannot be used as a measure of the health of a population, except in those situations in which access to health services and illness behaviour patterns are believed to be the same for everyone.

MEASURES OF FUNCTIONING

The problem with comparing the many different diagnoses likely to be discovered in a community prevalence study is that different diseases cause different degrees of incapacity, and even the same disease might be found with different stages of severity. One way around this problem is to ignore the specific diagnosis and instead measure the degree of incapacity produced by the illness; in this way, a case of heart disease can be compared with a case of arthritis through finding out to what extent the disease prevents the patient from carrying out his or her normal routine.

Measures of functioning have particularly been used in surveys of chronic illness when the disease has a specific impact on daily living. For this reason, these are often called activities of daily living (ADL) measures (Katz et al. 1963). An ADL measure identifies certain everyday functions, sometimes divided into major and minor, that are then assessed by means of a survey. For example, major items might include activities such as feeding oneself, getting to and using a toilet, and doing up buttons and zips. Minor items might include things like putting on shoes and socks, having a bath or wash, getting in and out of bed, combing and brushing hair. Respondents would be asked whether they can do any of these things, by themselves, with help or not at all (Harris 1971). Responses are then added up to create an overall score of disability. Such scores enable the amount of disability in a population to be measured.

The Disability Adjusted Life Years (DALY) incorporates measures of functioning into an overall population index. Thus, a disability measure is combined with the number of years that the disability is likely to be experienced (Murray and Lopez 1994). This means that incapacities occurring earlier in life contribute a greater weight to an overall population index than disabilities beginning in the elderly.

ADLs are said to be 'objective' measures because they enquire about activities that can easily be verified. Indeed, often it is the carer or health professional who answers on behalf of the patient, especially when the degree of incapacity is great. Yet in some ways this supposed objectivity is a weakness. This is not the patient's world, but that of the researcher who has decided that certain activities are important. But illness can affect people in many ways, not only in carrying out basic everyday activities. This view has led increasingly to a strategy of asking people themselves to make their own assessments of their health status.

SELF-REPORT MEASURES

One common measure of health is to ask people a simple, usually single, question about their health. In Britain, for example, the annual General Household Survey asks a sample of people about their experience of acute illness in the preceding 14 days and whether they believe they have a long-standing illness. These responses can then be summed to create measures of the acute or long-standing chronic illness in a population. More commonly, researchers ask respondents to rate their current health as excellent, good, fair or poor. Although a very simple question, the responses have been found to be an important predictor of subsequent mortality (Idler and Benyamin 1997).

Self-reported illness is relatively easy to measure but suffers from certain serious disadvantages.

- From the illness behaviour literature, it is known that some people are more likely to take their illnesses to the doctor than others. This same bias may also operate when reporting illness to an interviewer. Thus more 'stoical' people may report lower levels of illness, whereas others may exaggerate it.
- It is also known from research into illness behaviour that it is not simply the readiness to report illness that varies between people, but also their very perception of illness itself. Thus two people with exactly the same illness may perceive their health in different ways.

Even so, these 'biases' in the supposed accuracy of simple self-report measures may themselves be components of the broad range of predictive factors that make the association with later mortality so high.

SUBJECTIVE HEALTH MEASURES

Part of the limitation of self-reported sickness is the crudity of the measure: people are simply asked whether they have had an illness or not or whether they see themselves as healthy. A different approach is to use a more comprehensive questionnaire to enquire after health status. Because such questionnaires rely on the respondents' own view of their health, the measures are called subjective health indicators.

There are two broad approaches to creating a subjective health measure. One is to aim for a questionnaire that will produce a single global score (or index) of health status. This is particularly useful when comparing individuals or populations in that it can be clearly established whether one group has more 'health' than another. However, critics point out that health is multi-dimensional and something like mobility cannot be equated with, say, sleep. They therefore propose using health profiles that will give any individual a number of scores based on the number of dimensions of health measured in the questionnaire. Examples of the latter are the Nottingham Health Profile (NHP: Hunt et al. 1986), the Sickness Impact Profile (SIP: de Bruin et al. 1992) and the Short Form 36-item questionnaire (SF-36: Ware et al. 1986).

The NHP was developed by asking many people what they thought was important about good health. From their responses, a series of questions was devised that takes the form of 'I have pain at night', 'I find it hard to bend', 'Things are getting me down' and simply requires a yes/no response. These different questions are then grouped into the following six categories or dimensions of health:

- pain
- physical mobility
- sleep
- energy
- social isolation
- emotional reactions.

Another popular health profile, the SF-36, was developed from large-scale studies in the USA. It contains 36 questions that produce eight dimensions, namely:

- physical functioning
- social functioning
- role limitations due to physical problems
- role limitations due to emotional problems
- general mental health
- energy/vitality
- bodily pain
- general health perceptions.

The SF-36 is supposed to take only 5–10 minutes to complete and its exponents argue that it is more sensitive than the NHP to minor illness disturbances.

While the search for a single health status index is proving elusive, no doubt on account of the complexity of the idea of 'good health', multi-dimensional health profiles seem the best way forward. Medical treatments have traditionally been evaluated in terms of the biological changes in the patient's body resulting from medical intervention. Thus, giving iron to an anaemic woman is supposed to increase the haemoglobin level; giving antibiotics for lobar pneumonia improves the appearance on the chest X-ray and lung function. The advantage of subjective health measures is that the subjective responses of the patients themselves can be added to these biological parameters. Thus they can be used in:

- regular monitoring of patient care,
- improving doctor–patient interactions by informing doctors of the subjective well-being of their patients,
- clinical trials when evaluating two or more different treatments,
- assessing health gains in different patient groups, especially when considering 'best buys' in providing services (see Chapter 13),
- monitoring the health of the population.

QUALITY OF LIFE MEASURES

Another way of looking at health is to say that illness has an effect in terms of detracting from the quality of life. Why not, therefore, measure the quality of life directly? This can be particularly useful when assessing the value of medical intervention: a patient might not be cured, but some amelioration, even if slight, of the underlying condition is often an important factor in deciding whether to use the treatment another time (Clark and Fallowfield 1986).

There are many measures of quality of life available (Hollandsworth 1988; Bowling 1991), though their emphases differ and many, understandably, overlap considerably with so-called subjective health measures (as described above). Early measures tended to tap 'objective' facets of the quality of life – often defined by professional health care workers – whereas recent measures have tended to emphasize 'subjective' components more. The measures usually try to embrace both functional impairment and psychological well-being, and in this respect are often similar to a combined ADL and psychiatric morbidity measure.

Arguments continue as to the respective merits of different ways of measuring quality of life, but there is broad agreement that the idea of this measure is a good one in that ultimately all medical care – life-saving, curative, ameliorative and supportive – is somehow directed towards improving the quality of life of patients.

Assessment of quality of life has often arisen in situations in which it is important to evaluate 'value for money' in health service provision (see Chapter 13). These quality of life measures are often therefore combined with some sort of economic assessment to determine whether certain treatments are worthwhile in terms of the overall benefits they confer. For example, Quality Adjusted Life Years (QALYs) are calculated by combining the gain in life expectancy with a measure of the expected quality of life of those extra years (in this case using anticipated disability and distress), and then comparing the number of QALYs achieved against the cost of different treatments (Williams 1985). Further details about how QALYS are calculated and their role in determining health care provision are given in Chapter 13.

Yet, as with any subjective measure, there is always the argument that the chosen criteria of 'health' or 'good quality' are not appropriate for a particular patient. The next step, therefore, was to construct a measure that allowed patients not only allowed to express their opinion on quality of life but also to choose the criteria themselves, the so-called Schedule for the Evaluation of Individual Quality of Life (SEIQoL). Thus, patients start by listing several areas of their lives that are important to them – gardening, being pain free, family relationships etc. – and then these chosen areas are rated from good to bad and the different scores added. Later, patients can assess the same criteria, and comparison with their early responses should show whether or not there has been improvement. This whole process is rather cumbersome, but it does produce a quality of life score that is meaningful for that particular person (Hickey et al. 1996).

HEALTH AND EXPECTATIONS

It has been noted that in some countries in which health status has improved in recent decades – as indicated by declining (especially infant) mortality – subjective health assessments seem to have got worse, the so-called 'paradox of health' (Barsky 1988). The most likely explanation is that when health improves, expectations rise even faster, so that an 'objective' improvement is accompanied by a 'subjective' decline. In India, for example, the state of Kerala has the highest levels of literacy and longevity but it also has the highest rate of reported morbidity among all Indian states. The state of Bihar, on the other hand, has low longevity (and poor medical and educational facilities) but also the lowest rates of reported morbidity in India (Sen 2002). The comparison can be extended to the USA, where reported illness is even greater than in Kerala, despite much better 'objective' health indices.

It has also been observed that sometimes patients with severe and progressive chronic illness report improving quality of life over time: how can this happen? Again, it is likely to be due to changing expectations. As the impact of illness sinks in, patients come to value new things and recalibrate their assessments, with the result that they cope better with the limitations inflicted by the illness (and produce a 'response shift' in the answers to the quality of life measure (Sprangers and Schwartz 1999).

These observations about the importance of expectations in relation to how people perceive their health are significant in understanding two major phenomena in health care. One is the ever-increasing demands made on health care despite apparently continually improving health status. The other is the way in which patients so frequently cope (or sometimes fail to cope) with serious debilitating illness. Understanding the role of patients' expectations is clearly an important part of explaining the demand for and use of health care in the twenty-first century. In this sense, it is not the state of the biological body that is important, but rather the accompanying patient's psychosocial perspective.

MEASURING HEALTH

The measurement of health in different ways produces different assessments of how healthy someone is. Sometimes these measures are closely related, and sometimes they produce quite different perspectives – for example physiological assessments of 'fitness' seem to bear little relationship to psychosocial health as measured by questionnaire (Blaxter 1990). The measurement of these different notions of health and illness is clearly important and the technical issues are well discussed elsewhere (Culyer 1983; McDowell and Newell 1987; Fallowfield 1990; Bowling 1991, 1995). From the simple but crude measure of the mortality rate, to the more subtle changes of subjective health status, assessments of health are deemed increasingly important in evaluating medical treatments and in making decisions about the provision of health care. These different measures of health also give a flavour of the wide variety of ways that health can be construed and these have significance in the examination of particular causes, patterns and effects of illness, as covered in succeeding chapters.

Chapter 4

SOCIAL CAUSES
OF ILLNESS

Textbooks of pathology and clinical medicine describe factors that cause disease. The descriptions are dominated by the biomedical model of illness in which a biological change is seen as being brought about by a preceding biological change. Sociology offers three challenges to this perspective:

1 the presence of many biological causes of illness is strongly influenced by social factors;
2 illness is multi-dimensional – a description of the causes of the biological lesion alone is not an adequate explanation if that illness has psychosocial dimensions that equally need understanding;
3 there is evidence that apparently biologically based diseases, and even death, may be directly brought about by social factors.

CAUSAL MODELS

Before exploring the role of social factors in the aetiology of illness, it is important to clarify the notion of cause. Put simply, if a change in one variable brings about change in another, then the former can be said to cause the latter. This can be expressed in notation as:

$$A \rightarrow B$$

where A is the cause and B the effect. Examples abound in clinical medicine: a virus causes influenza, a fall causes a fracture, atheroma causes coronary heart disease, etc.

However, for almost all diseases, this model is an abstraction in that the actual causal system is known to be far more complex. At the simplest level, the supposed causal relationship between A and B ignores why A changes, and it ignores the possible 'mechanisms' by which A changes B. Thus a more comprehensive model might be:

$$x \rightarrow A \rightarrow y \rightarrow B$$

A and *B* are still causally related, but so are *x* and *B*, and *y* and *B*. The answer to the question 'What causes *B*?' can now be provided in three ways, all different but all correct.

Sometimes in medicine, apparently alternative explanations are merely different selections from the same causal sequence. For example, it is argued later that social class is incriminated in the aetiology of many diseases such as infections and heart disease, yet medical textbooks are more likely to stress bacteria and serum cholesterol levels. How can these two apparently different sets of explanations be reconciled?

The two explanations, the biological and the social, are not necessarily in conflict if they are taken from different points in the same causal sequence. Thus, it may be that:

$$\text{low social class} \rightarrow \text{poor diet} \rightarrow \text{high serum cholesterol} \rightarrow$$
$$\text{coronary heart disease}$$

In which case, both biological and social explanations are correct.

The picture in medicine is further complicated by the fact that disease aetiology cannot properly be represented by such a simple causal sequence; instead a multifactorial model is more appropriate.

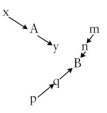

For example, for a patient to develop tuberculosis may require both the presence of the bacillus and a poor nutritional state (which might be a product of social conditions). Hence both factors may be necessary pre-conditions for developing the disease.

In medicine, when the cause of a disease is identified, it represents a choice from a wide selection of possible causal factors, both in type and over time. As the environment is a factor in the causation of most diseases, and the social environment is inextricably intertwined in the biological/physical, most diseases have some social factors bound up in their aetiology, as is argued later in this chapter.

ESTABLISHING A CAUSAL RELATIONSHIP

There are three conditions that must be fulfilled for it to be possible to claim that two variables are causally related, e.g. *A* causes *B* ($A \rightarrow B$).

1 They must occur in the correct *temporal sequence*: the independent variable, *A*, must precede the dependent variable, *B*, in time; if it does not, their rela-

tionship cannot be causal. In the natural sciences, discovering the temporal sequence of two variables may be relatively easy, especially in a laboratory when the timing of interventions can be controlled. However, in the social and behavioural sciences, and especially under non-experimental conditions, it may be difficult. For instance, there is some suggestion that being made redundant is a high risk for becoming depressed, but equally plausible would be the hypothesis that depression tends to lead to job loss through an inability to work properly.

2 There must be a *correlation* between the variables such that as *A* varies, *B* varies (*A* %; *B*). In other words, there should be a dose–response relationship. It is customary to use statistical tests to show such co-variation.

3 There must be *no third explanatory variable*. This is the most difficult condition to exclude. If a third variable exists that affects both *A* and *B*, the observed relationship between the latter may be spurious.

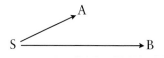

For instance, there may be a correlation between the number of television sets and heart attacks in the population:

number of television sets % heart attacks

However, it is unlikely that one is causing the other. By introducing a third variable, affluence, a more plausible model is produced: affluence causes increased spending on consumer goods and the sale of televisions increases; at the same time, affluence produces a change in lifestyle, perhaps in diet, that may increase the heart attack rate. Thus:

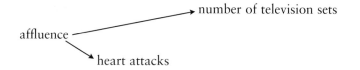

The apparent relationship between numbers of television sets and heart attacks is therefore spurious as it is explained by the third variable, affluence.

A more familiar example is that of the relationship between cigarette smoking and lung cancer. There is a well-established correlation between these two variables and they occupy the correct temporal sequence (it seems highly unlikely that having lung cancer makes a patient smoke cigarettes). But is the relationship causal?

It was once suggested that it is a personality type that 'causes' both cigarette smoking and cancer. Thus it is possible to construct two different causal models to show the relationship between smoking and lung cancer.

(i)   smoking $\rightarrow$ cancer

(ii)   extraversion $\nearrow$ smoking $\searrow$ cancer

In both models, there is the correct temporal sequence and both models will show a correlation between smoking and cancer. A test of the latter hypothesis became available when one section of the population (doctors) radically decreased their cigarette consumption after a link between smoking and cancer was first suggested. The result was a decrease in cancer in this group. If the second model had been correct, stopping smoking should have had no effect on their cancer rate, because personalities, which supposedly caused the cancer, remained constant.

However, even though in this study the hypothesized causal relationship between smoking and cancer was confirmed, it does not prevent other 'third' variables from surfacing to challenge an established relationship. For instance, doctors' cancer rate may have gone down not because they gave up smoking, but because they also perhaps became less anxious and it is anxious people who get cancer and who tend to smoke.

In other words, the condition for causality that specifies the absence of a third variable (that shows the apparent relationship to be spurious) is unattainable. However, this does not mean that the hypothesized relationship should be rejected; it is at least now known that smoking is a better explanation of the cause of cancer than extraversion. The claim of causality therefore is always a provisional one. It is only by successive testing of the relationship against the more obvious and plausible alternatives that increased reliance can be placed on the hypothesis linking two variables despite its inherently provisional nature.

SOCIAL FACTORS: INDIRECT EFFECTS

Medicine has identified many risk factors that increase the chances that an individual will become ill or even die. Smoking, diet, genetics etc. can all be used to estimate a risk profile for an individual patient (see also Chapter 9). There can, however, be too much emphasis on individual risk factors and not enough on the social context from which many of these individualized risks emerge and to which health care interventions might more appropriately be directed (Link and Phelan 1995).

The role of social context in the cause of illness can be seen in two ways. There can be an indirect effect in which social factors bring the individual and a harmful physical/biological agent together in some way. For example, although it may be water-borne organisms that cause an illness, it is the particular social customs of a community in drinking from a stream or from a well that will help determine their disease patterns. Alternatively, social factors may have a direct effect through which something in the social environment triggers an illness without any apparent physical intermediary.

Given the multi-factorial aetiology of most diseases, it is probable that both indirect and direct effects are involved together in many illnesses; however, for purposes of description they are dealt with separately here. First, the evidence for the influence of social factors in bringing hazards from the physical/biological world into contact with people is described. These influences can be seen as either general or specific.

GENERAL INFLUENCE OF SOCIAL FACTORS

Dubos (1980) argued that illness was a product of environmental maladaptation. He suggested societies that had reached an equilibrium with their natural environment were, by and large, disease free, disease only arising when that balance was disturbed. In the age of colonialism, immunologically unprotected populations were wiped out by the disastrous spread of European endemic infections such as measles. However, more relevant for Western society is the speed of social change with industrialization and its aftermath. According to Dubos, this continuous change produced disequilibrium and maladaptation to the environment. This in its turn produced illness. For example, if all change in diet were to stop, then those individuals who were harmed by certain foods would have an evolutionary disadvantage and gradually, over time, their genes would be lost; eventually there would be a society without diet-induced illness as everyone would be adapted to the society's foodstuffs. In other words, the price of a healthy society, according to Dubos, would be one in which change, whatever its form, was stopped and replaced by stability.

SPECIFIC INFLUENCE OF SOCIAL FACTORS

The second and more common way of looking at the effect of the natural environment on people is to see it in terms of specific hazards. McKeown (1979) argued that the high mortality rate in the nineteenth century – and, by implication, in developing countries today – was the product of micro-organism-based diseases that flourished in a setting of insanitary conditions and poor nutrition. One of the specific examples he provided was the decline in mortality from tuberculosis from the middle of the nineteenth century when the causes of death were first recorded to the late twentieth century. Although one of the important aetiological factors in tuberculosis, the tubercle bacillus, was discovered in the late nineteenth century, it was not until 1948 that a specific treatment (streptomycin) was available. Nevertheless, by 1948, over 90 per cent of the decline in mortality from the disease had already occurred. The explanation that McKeown advanced for this phenomenon was the improvement in sanitation and nutrition that occurred during the nineteenth and early twentieth centuries. McKeown calculated that similar factors have been at work since the nineteenth century for most causes of death and, at most, medical intervention (mainly since the Second World War) accounted for only about 4 per cent of the total improvement in life expectancy over the succeeding century and a half (see Figure 4.1).

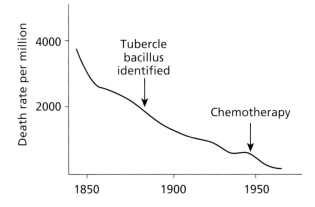

Figure 4.1 Decline in mortality from tuberculosis (after McKeown 1979).

Although sanitary conditions in modern society have been transformed, virtually eliminating water-borne diseases, and the nutritional state of the population has risen to such an extent that host resistance is much improved, environmental factors such as pollution, work hazards, poor diet etc. are no doubt still important in the aetiology of many diseases. Indeed, it is not only current living conditions that play a role in disease aetiology, but also conditions in the past. There is now evidence to suggest that adult diseases such as hypertension, ischaemic heart disease, stroke and chronic bronchitis may be determined by *in utero* and early childhood experiences, especially in terms of nutrition – the so-called Fetal Origins Hypothesis (Barker 1992; Kuh and Wadsworth 1993).

Although each of the above environmental physical/biological factors is important in the aetiology of disease, all of these factors occur in a social context. As McKeown pointed out, improvements in nutrition have not necessarily been consciously brought about, but have reflected the improving standard of living of the population at large. Equally, the battles fought by sanitary reformers in the nineteenth century (often against orthodox medicine) show that the socio-political will must also be present to introduce adequate environmental safeguards. Pollution and occupational hazards also relate to individual behaviour and group interests – and, of course, cigarette smoking, the largest avoidable cause of mortality in developed countries, is very much a behaviour that influences health.

McKeown provided data on the improvement in life expectancy by age group and whether smokers or not. Figure 4.2 shows that the improvement in life expectancy over 130 years was at least halved in each age group by the simple behaviour of smoking. Put another way, half of all the improvements, whether brought about by nutrition, sanitation, housing, standard of living, or medical therapeutics, were eliminated by a single behaviour. This illustrates most powerfully the importance of belief and behaviour as risk factors in the bringing together of hazardous chemicals and the individual human body.

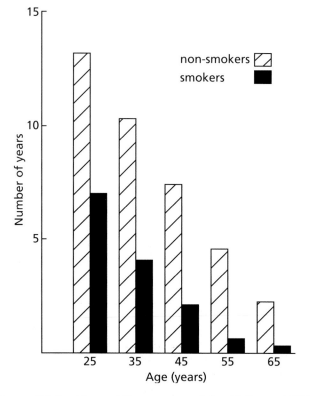

Figure 4.2 Smoking and life expectancy (after McKeown 1979).

SOCIAL FACTORS: DIRECT EFFECTS

Specific environmental hazards such as cigarette smoke or unclean water can clearly damage cellular structure to such a degree as to produce clinical disease. It is, perhaps, less easy to see how a non-physical 'hazard' can bring about a similar process. Even so, at times diseases seem to arise independently of any physical factor. In addition, taking a wider definition of health that embraces subjective response and quality of life as well as physical abnormality, it is apparent that non-physical influences play a major role in ill-health. Medicine sometimes refers to diseases without an organic cause as 'functional'; sometimes such illnesses have been called psychosomatic in that there appears to be a direct effect of the mind on the body.

Is more difficult to demonstrate the role of non-physical hazards than the place of physical insult in the aetiology of illness. There are a number of reasons for this and, before summarizing the field, it may be helpful to identify some of the problems that researchers must tackle in attempting to establish a firm link between social factors and ill-health, in whatever form.

METHODOLOGICAL DIFFICULTIES

- To show a relationship between, say, stress and ill-health, it would be necessary to measure both variables and see if they correlate. To allow for the influence of other factors, it is customary to establish an equivalent control group that does not experience the threat and whose rate of illness is then compared with the experimental group. Such research designs can immediately create problems because natural experiments in which a random half of a population is stressed and the other half is not stressed are hard to find. It may be possible to replicate stress in the laboratory, but there must then be doubts about its relevance and applicability to the world outside.
- There are difficulties in measuring ill-health that have already been outlined in Chapter 3. Mortality is relatively easy to measure, but many of the effects of psychosocial factors are believed to be forms of ill-health that are less specific and definite.
- The social factor itself must also be measured. For example, in measuring stress, the researcher must decide what stress actually is. The problem is that different researchers often define it in different ways, resulting in different forms of measurement and, hence, studies that are not directly comparable.
- Finally, it is often difficult to distinguish between the social factor and ill-health in the measurement process. A researcher trying to answer the question of whether stress causes depression might ask if someone is having difficulty sleeping as an indicator of whether they are under pressure and stressed; but, in addition, insomnia might be used as an indicator of clinical depression. There is obviously something circular about this argument: a person with depression might well seem to be stressed if stress is measured in a way similar to that of depression.

Some of the above difficulties illustrate the problems in showing the effect of social influences on a person's health. This means that studies in this area need to be viewed particularly critically. (It seems ironic that some biomedical scientists have been known to refer to the social sciences as 'soft sciences'; if anything, a social scientist must show more care in carrying out research or in evaluating such studies than might be expected in many natural science experiments.)

Notwithstanding these methodological difficulties, researchers have shown that non-physical factors seem to have an effect through two different mechanisms. One is the idea of a direct insult, as in a stressful event such as a bereavement. It is clear that such traumas can precipitate psychological disturbance and sometimes physical illness. But perhaps of more interest is the role of social factors in affecting someone's vulnerability or, conversely, their resistance to illness. This idea has led to a theory of a general susceptibility to illness (Cassel 1976), but has been most developed in ideas of the effect of social support. The rest of this chapter examines these ideas in terms of the four interrelated notions of social integration, social support, social capital and life events; the next chapter looks at the other major approach to direct social aetiology, namely labelling.

SOCIAL INTEGRATION

Social integration played a major role in the theory of social development advanced by the great sociologist Emile Durkheim at the end of the nineteenth century (Durkheim 1933). Durkheim argued that pre-industrial societies were characterized by such strong social bonds that individualism was submerged – what was important was the well-being of the social group. With the advent of industrialization and a division of labour (which divided work tasks into more and more specialized parts), social integration based on a common purpose and identity weakened and changed. Instead, social cohesion became based on a belief in individuality and it was the interdependence of people that held a society together.

The shift from a cohesive community based on strong social integration to a more amorphous and loosely structured society does not necessarily go smoothly. On the one hand, if social integration becomes too weak, individuals will be endangered by their isolation; on the other hand, if a new individualized identity fails to replace the former community identity, the individual is said to suffer from anomie, a sort of normlessness in which identity and sense of purpose become lost.

In a major study of suicide in Europe in the late nineteenth century, Durkheim applied his social theory to explore what might be regarded as the ultimate individual act, namely suicide (Durkheim 1952). He argued that despite its apparent solitary nature, suicide was underpinned by fundamentally social processes. He predicted four different types of suicide (Table 4.1). In pre-industrial societies, or in those communities in modern society that deny or repress individuality, two forms of suicide are produced. Altruistic suicide occurs when the death results from an over-integration of the individual in the social group such that concern for others overweighs personal interest: examples might be a soldier who dies for his colleagues, or a disabled member of the family who dies to relieve the burden on his or her relatives. Durkheim argued that fatalistic suicide, which was produced by over-regulation, was relatively rare, but one example was the ritualistic ceremony of *suti* in which Indian widows used to throw themselves on to their husbands' funeral pyres.

With the break-up of traditional community and its close interpersonal ties – to be replaced by the weaker bonds of modern society – the predominant sorts of suicide become dominated by under-regulation and under-integration. Thus,

Table 4.1 Durkheim's four types of suicide

	Too much	Too little
Social integration	Altruistic	Egoistic
Social regulation	Fatalistic	Anomic

After Durkheim (1952).

Durkheim argued, in modern society people mainly commit suicide because they are too isolated or because they feel their life lacks purpose and meaning.

In industrial and post-industrial society, in which under-integration and under-regulation are the primary hazards, any form of social bonding should, in principle, protect against suicide. Durkheim explored this possibility by examining situations in which individuals were socially isolated. For example, he reasoned that by stressing individual redemption, Protestants were less integrated into their religious community than Catholics or Jews and should therefore, according to his theory, show a higher rate of suicide. Equally, single people, widows and widowers should show a higher rate than otherwise similarly positioned married people. Also he suggested that the social integration produced by a common enemy during war should produce lower suicide rates than peacetime. And, when he examined European suicide data for the period, he found these various hypotheses confirmed.

Although Durkheim's work was carried out more than a century ago, his findings and explanations for variation in suicide rates still hold today. But, more importantly, his insights have been extended to other forms of illness, particularly the influence of poor social integration on health. It has been argued that social cohesiveness provides a major influence on the health of a population and that threats to that sense of integration such as large income disparities result in worse health for everyone (Wilkinson 1996). One way of thinking about the cohesive nature of a community is in terms of its 'social capital' (see below).

SOCIAL SUPPORT

Drawing on Durkheim's original hypotheses, modern researchers have tried to examine the relationship between social support and illness. The argument is that an important indicator of degree of social integration is the amount of social support someone may have, and this in its turn may determine his or her susceptibility to illness.

MARRIAGE AS SUPPORT

Modern suicide rates confirm, as in Durkheim's day, the value of social support insofar as single, widowed and divorced (still) people have higher rates than those who are married. Further, it is also apparent that the single, widowed and divorced also tend to have higher mortality rates in general when compared with married people. For some illnesses, the differences are quite striking. Table 4.2 shows the relative risk of dying for a number of different causes of death (Joung et al. 1996).

These are, however, broad brush strokes. Marital status might be related to mortality rates, but there are various possible alternative explanations for this finding that do not involve a direct influence of social support.

Table 4.2 Marital status and relative risk of mortality (Netherlands 1986–1990)

	Married	Single	Widowed	Divorced
Men				
Total mortality	1.0	1.47	1.28	1.62
Cancers	1.0	1.05	1.13	1.23
Diabetes	1.0	1.92	1.51	2.17
Injury and poisoning	1.0	2.92	2.09	3.82
Women				
Total mortality	1.0	1.24	1.23	1.49
Cancers	1.0	1.16	1.12	1.26
Diabetes	1.0	0.83	1.35	1.40
Injury and poisoning	1.0	2.32	1.90	2.99

After Joung et al. (1996).

- Single, never married, people may start off being more ill – perhaps that is why they failed to marry.
- Widowed people may have been subjected to the same environmental hazards as their spouses and therefore be more at risk for this reason
- Divorced people, because of their situation, may deliberately engage in hazardous activities.

It may be possible, therefore, to explain the link between marital status and mortality without recourse to a direct effect of social support itself. Nevertheless, as with any scientific explanation, a single cause is more elegant than proposing three different ones. The suspicion thus remains that it is one factor, namely social support, that links together these excesses of mortality in unmarried people. The search has continued to identify the specific links between social support and ill-health.

CONTACTS AS SOCIAL SUPPORT

Researchers in the area of social support faced some of the methodological problems described earlier in this chapter. First, what is actually meant by social support? How is it to be defined? Second, what is the best measure of ill-health that is most likely to show a relationship with social support?

In early studies, social support was defined in terms of number of interpersonal contacts. Thus, a person with 20 contacts a week had twice the social support of a person with ten contacts. A major long-term investigation in the USA, the Alameda County Study, reported that after allowing for other known factors in the cause of death, the extent of a person's social network corresponded to his or her risk of early mortality (Berkman and Syme 1979). The study's measure of social network was an amalgam of various aspects of social contact, and critics could argue that it was somehow constructed to fit the mortality data. Corroborative evidence, however, came from another study (Schoenbach et al. 1986), though in this case the size of networks seemed only linked to protection for white males.

QUALITY OF SUPPORT

The problem of measuring number of contacts as an indicator of social support is that it is possible that the actual numbers are not important. A person could converse with 50 different people in a day, yet none of them may be important or close enough to provide support; moreover, some social ties could be a source of strain. On the other hand, one close friend may be of great worth. This argument led to various studies that have tried to measure the quality of contacts as well as their number (Henderson 1980).

SUPPORT AS PERCEPTION

Attempts to measure the quality of supporting relationships led to the idea that perhaps 'quality' did not exist in the form of the relationship, but in the perception and expectations of the person being supported. In other words, friends might not actually be offering any support but, if the person believes that they are – or that they would if called upon – then this should have the same psychological impact as if there was support present. In short, it was not the social support itself but the belief in the social support that was important.

If social support is simply the belief in its existence, people with strong beliefs should be more protected from illness than those without. A particular example of this is religious belief in which the person has the perceived support of both a spiritual deity and the religious community to which he or she belongs. Moreover, religion can also be beneficial in cultivating attitudes that give the individual a helpful perspective in facing stressful situations. This latter would accord with Durkheim's observation that suicides are less common in religious groups that emphasize their sense of community. However, research into the effects of religious belief is made difficult by the fact that many religions often recommend certain types of behaviour that might, quite independently, be protective for the individual.

The evidence linking lowered mortality with religious affiliation is limited, mainly because religion is not usually placed on the death certificate in most countries. Even so, it has been shown that certain religious groups probably benefit from proscription of some potentially harmful behaviours. For example, Seventh Day Adventists are a religious group who abstain from alcohol, tobacco, beverages containing caffeine and from certain meats and, probably as a result, have a longer life expectancy compared with the rest of the population. Equally, Mormons are proscribed certain foods, as well as smoking, and they too seem to have longer life expectancy and lower incidences of certain diseases. In fact, it has been suggested that much of the variation observed in mortality between religious groups can be explained by cigarette smoking alone.

In studies of the effects of religion on various aspects of health and illness, it is mostly religious affiliation that has been measured, and not the religious belief. Yet, from the previous discussion of social support, it seems that the belief – and therefore perception of support – may be the more important variable. There is some evidence to support the view that commitment to a religion, measured in terms of church attendance, does contribute to better health (Hannay 1980). However, there may be a selection effect such that those who feel ill participate less extensively in religious activities than those who feel well.

Other studies also suggest an important influence of religious commitment on social support and health. The Alameda County Study (Berkman and Syme 1979) showed that church attendance was related to low mortality, though church attendance was simply one component of a wider social network. Another study (Kasl and Ostfield 1984) examined 400 elderly poor for their religiousness and mortality. They found that church attendance and self-rated religiousness both seemed to have an effect on decreasing mortality, suggesting that the effect of religion was probably not only due to social contacts.

The idea that social support might protect people from illness and death remains a fascinating one and, despite the measurement difficulties, it is important that further studies try to untangle this no doubt important influence on health status.

SOCIAL CAPITAL

Another way of thinking about a social support network is to see it as a fixed resource or form of capital. Just as someone's financial capital in terms of money in the bank can be seen as a resource that will afford some protection against challenges to their material well-being, so social capital may protect against the life threats that people experience. However, because social capital is defined in terms of the social networks in which an individual is embedded, it can also – and probably better – be looked at as a characteristic of a community rather than of an individual. In other words, social capital is shared, as, by definition, one individual cannot have social capital if neighbours do not. Thus, a community with high social capital will have strong social ties and mutual trust.

Social capital does seem to offer some protection against wider social ills. For example, it has been argued that communities with high social capital have better mental health and are more crime free than those without (Putnam 2000). In addition, there does seem to be a good relationship between social capital and measures of health such as mortality (Kawachi et al. 1997). The idea of social capital seems a useful one in bringing together the classic work of Durkheim on the importance of social integration with the major intangible effects that cohesiveness and social support seem to have on everyone's health (Berkman et al. 2000), and it allows the more intangible aspects of the wider social environment to be seen in their relationship to illness (McCulloch 2001).

LIFE EVENTS

It has been observed over many years that a negative life event such as a bereavement is likely to precipitate a reaction that resembles clinical depression. This has led researchers to suggest that negative life events, like the loss of bereavement, may be important in the aetiology of other illnesses.

Early attempts to measure life events used a checklist format in which respondents had simply to tick if any particular event had happened to them in a certain time period (Holmes and Rahe 1967). These events were then weighted by the researchers according to their assessment of severity, and the resulting values were summed to give an overall life event score. In recent years, it has been argued that this technique is too crude because it fails to take into account the particular meanings of events for different people. For example, for most people, the death of an elderly parent is a negative and traumatic event, but for some it may be a release from a very strained and difficult situation. It is therefore important to know the context of the event before rating its degree of threat for the individual.

Most work on the influence of life events in the aetiology of disease has concentrated on psychiatric disorder (Dohrenwend and Dohrenwend 1981). Whereas it was known that the death of a close friend or relative produced a bereavement reaction with close similarities to depression, the bereavement reaction was believed to be a normal event, which tended to be self-limiting. Depression was a clinical syndrome, however, that continued beyond a reasonable time and, indeed, in many cases did not seem to be preceded by life events. Early work therefore concentrated on identifying to what extent episodes of clinical depression could be related to external negative life events.

Brown and his co-workers carried out an in-depth study of women in south London to examine the relationship between life events and depressive disorder (Brown and Harris 1978). They found a fairly clear relationship between experiencing a life event and the onset of depression, though the influence of the life event on the illness also seemed to depend on several other 'vulnerability' factors that might increase the susceptibility of the women in the study to becoming depressed. These factors were: no employment outside the home, the presence of children aged less than 5 at home, lack of a good intimate relationship with someone, and the death of the woman's own mother before the age of 11. The model they proposed was therefore multi-factorial, but it meant that if the vulnerability risk factors were all stacked against a woman, a life event became much more likely to tip her into depression. For example, for working-class women with young children at home in a poor marriage, the risk of clinical depression was almost 50 per cent. It might be added that much of the depression brought about by life events identified in the study had not been presented to the health service.

In an extension to the south London study, Brown and his co-workers looked at the prevalence of psychiatric disorder on the Hebridean island of North Uist (Brown et al. 1977). They found that while the overall amount of psychiatric morbidity on the island was not dissimilar to that found in the London study, the type of illness was different. Whereas in London almost all the morbidity had been depression, on North Uist there was a considerable amount of anxiety as well. (Most depressive disorder has anxiety components and vice versa; in most cases, however, a major component can be identified.)

The interesting feature of the distribution of depression and anxiety in North Uist was its relationship to social integration. Those women who were closely integrated into the traditional community on the island (those born on the island, working in traditional industries such as crofting and fishing, and closely linked to the church) were more likely to suffer from anxiety, whereas the others, like the Camberwell women, were more likely to suffer from depression. This finding resonated with Durkheim's original observations of the protective features of social integration and social support. Brown speculated that the integrated women were only experiencing psychiatric disorder because their traditional way of life was changing rapidly with the new oil industry and growing tourism. This made their traditional security seem precarious and produced an anxiety reaction.

There have since been several attempts to establish a link between life events and organic disease (Creed 1985). There seems to be some support for the influence of life events on subarachnoid haemorrhage, myocardial infarction and functional abdominal pain as well as on patients presenting illness without identifiable pathology (Katon et al. 2001). One study involving patients with appendicitis showed an interesting link between abdominal pain and life (Creed 1981). All the patients in the sample were asked about preceding life events; these events were grouped into two types, threatening (that could happen) and severe (that had actually occurred). Pathology reports on the removed appendix were then examined. These showed, as is usual, that about half the appendices removed were not pathologically inflamed. However, when the pathology report was related to the experience of life events, it was found that those patients with severe events were more likely to have a non-inflamed appendix.

It is clear that life events and social support are related, but there is some debate as to the connection. One view is that social support has an influence on illness quite independent of life events – though often the two can be additive. The other view is that social support offers a 'buffer' for life events in which the negative impact of an event is somehow reduced by good social support. For example, a study of social support in physically disabled people found that low social support was associated with significant deterioration in psychosocial and emotional functioning only in the presence of adverse life events (Patrick et al. 1986). On the other hand, a life event can itself undermine social support: for example, an infant death has a negative impact on the quality of the relationship between its grieving parents (Najman et al. 1993).

Many studies have now shown the value of careful methodological work in the elucidation of the role of life events in illness. Debates continue as to the best method of measuring life events and their precise relationship with social support, but there can be little doubt that they play a significant role in people's sense of well-being.

Chapter 5

LABELLING BEHAVIOUR

One of the theories of how life events make their impact is through a person's sense of self-esteem. Day-to-day interaction can be looked upon as requiring so much self-esteem, but when that self-esteem is threatened, such as by a life event, then people are less able to cope and manifest signs of psychological disturbance. Another important way in which self-esteem might be challenged is through 'labelling'.

Labelling refers to the process whereby individual characteristics are identified by others and given a negative label (Lemert 1967). This process involves judgements about what is socially normal/acceptable and what is abnormal/deviant. The height of someone taken from the tail of a normal population distribution is 'abnormal' to the extent that it, say, lies outside two standard deviations of the mean, but it is only 'deviant' if it is in some way held to be socially abnormal. Startlingly blue eyes may be remarked upon as unusual but the person is unlikely to be cast as deviant, unlike, perhaps, the albino whose eye colour is both unusual and socially strange. Deviance therefore implies some degree of negative social evaluation.

But why is it that of two unusual eye colours one is viewed as deviant and the other is not? Why is it that a man who talks to himself in church is praying, while a man who talks to himself in the street is mad? 'Labelling theory', as it is often called, has been developed to help answer these questions. It is divided between two notions of deviance, primary and secondary.

PRIMARY DEVIANCE

The concept of primary deviance relates to the actual defining of a state or behaviour as 'deviant'. This is most easily seen in the passing of laws that make an act that was 'normal' become illegal or deviant, or, conversely, the 'decriminalization' of some behaviour, such as homosexuality, by a simple piece of legislation. Similarly, the act of diagnosis, of affixing disease labels to people, is a process of classification by which people are labelled ill (deviant) or healthy.

Labelling as a means of creating diseases should be distinguished from the cause of diseases. Bacteria cause disease, but also, acting in the gut as commensurals, they 'cause' health. Whether bacteria cause disease is therefore not an inherent property of the organism but rather a retrospective judgement based on whether the resulting physiopathological state is 'labelled' as disease or health. Diseases are labels, just as are the descriptions given any so-called deviant behaviour (see Chapter 14 for further discussion of this mechanism for 'creating' disease).

The labelling of primary deviance is important because it enables apparently similar phenomena to be separated into socially acceptable and unacceptable. A gang of working-class teenagers who break windows in a public building might be labelled as 'vandals', but a group of drunken medical students after a rugby game carrying out a similar act might be more likely to be showing 'high spirits'. Similarly, if a person claims with some conviction that he is Napoleon, it might be considered good acting if he is on the stage or schizophrenia if he is in the doctor's surgery. The behaviour in both instances may be virtually the same, but the social interpretation – and therefore the label – differs.

The labelling of primary deviance is therefore a means by which the normal is reaffirmed and the deviant is identified. Labelling in this sense serves to delineate the boundaries of what is considered to be normal social values and behaviour (Becker 1963). From this perspective, diagnosis is a process of identifying and labelling primary deviance that defines the bounds of social normality (see Chapter 13).

SECONDARY DEVIANCE

Secondary deviance refers to the change in behaviour that occurs as a consequence of labelling. Strong social pressures tend to promote behaviour in conformity with the label, and labelling thereby becomes a 'self-fulfilling prophecy' (Schur 1971).

STEREOTYPING

The pressures on patients to change their behaviour arise from the social meaning and significance of the label the doctor has applied. A blind person may be seen as quiet and docile, a psychiatric patient as dangerous, an epileptic patient as violent. These particular stereotypes may affect both patients' perception of themselves and the responses of those around them.

INTERPERSONAL INTERACTION

The interpersonal behaviour of a labelled person may be affected as people respond to him differently. This response, whether it is based on an attempt to ignore or help, can reaffirm the new self-image of the labelled person. Do people talk to the blind person on the bus in the same way that they talk with other people? Some people can become quite embarrassed when they suddenly discover that the person they were talking to at the table is paraplegic: what had they been saying? Had they inadvertently said things that may have shocked or hurt?

The response of so-called normal people to disability may be well meaning, but the result can often be to bring the behaviour of the person so labelled into conformity with people's expectations. There is some evidence, for example, of a 'halo' effect in the classroom such that if a teacher is told that certain children are intelligent, even if they are only of medium ability, the labelled children achieve better results than otherwise similar children.

RETROSPECTIVE INTERPRETATION

The other difference in behaviour towards people with so-called deviant attributes – particularly the mentally ill – is that there is often a search through the person's past life to find events and behaviour that will justify today's label. This process of 'retrospective interpretation' occurs in everyday interaction and is also commonly found in the media coverage of events. The suicide of an apparently contented public figure seems perplexing until past events, perhaps a bout of depression 5 years ago, make sense of the event. But do they? Most of the people who have had depression during the past 5 years do not commit suicide. And what of the last 4 years of contentment? The answer is that the present is comprehended and interpreted by reference to the past – if necessary, distorting the past to make it explain the present.

In many ways, a doctor's notes are distortions of past events because they are selective. They do not record when the patient did not have headaches or was very happy, only when the headaches occurred or when the patient was depressed. This is not to argue that the current basis of writing clinical notes is wrong, only to point out that one of the unintended consequences of this practice may be to reinforce in the doctor's mind the correctness of the current diagnosis.

RELEVANCE OF SECONDARY DEVIANCE TO MEDICINE

The notion of secondary deviance is of importance to medicine in that certain disease labels carry with them public stereotypes that may change a patient's behaviour. For example, a man fully recovered from a myocardial infarction may refuse to return to work and become a near-invalid, confined to the house, because of the image he and his family and friends have of the 'coronary cripple'. A diagnosed epileptic may refuse to go swimming or cross a busy road and may become depressed and withdrawn, again because of the social meaning placed on the diagnostic label.

In many cases, these consequences are almost unavoidable; it is only by giving the patient a diagnosis, whether it is blindness, epilepsy, sexually transmitted disease etc., that adequate treatment and care can be arranged for him or her. In other cases, the effect can be lessened if the doctor is aware of the potential effects the diagnosis might carry and therefore handles it more cautiously. In other words, a diagnosis is not simply a convenient classification given to some underlying biological phenomenon: it may also be a label that carries significant social meaning. To tell a patient she has Hashimoto's disease will probably draw a blank, but to tell a patient she is blind or a diabetic or an epileptic may well set in motion significant changes in her life as a direct consequence of the social meaning carried by the diagnosis (Scott 1969). In the end, these changes may have a greater effect on the patient's life than the biological dysfunction that was originally described.

STIGMA

The power of a label to bring about secondary deviance stems from social reaction to the person so labelled. But patients are also part of that same world of meaning and they too have similar reactions to their own diagnoses. Thus, both patient and others react to a diagnosis of 'heart disease' because of the general understanding of the meaning of the problem. There are therefore two components to the reaction to a diagnosis, that of the patient and that of others that may in turn impinge on the patient's own reaction.

For certain health problems it is not the specific medical diagnosis that brings out the social reaction, but the general visibility of the particular condition. A patient who cannot see or hear or walk can easily be identified by others without a formal medical diagnosis; and because such patients do not obviously possess all of the attributes of 'normal' people, they may be seen in some sense as socially unacceptable or inferior. People with such 'abnormalities' are said to be *stigmatized* (Goffman 1963).

People with stigmatized conditions are essentially outsiders: their stigma marks them out for social rejection. However, in terms of the impact of a label on the person, it is not only the social reaction that is important, but also the imagined social reaction. Many patients with epilepsy successfully conceal it from friends and relatives (and even their spouses) so there is no overt social reaction to the diagnosis; however, these patients can still experience 'felt stigma' in that they feel themselves to be inferior, to be hiding a discreditable part of their character from the world outside (Scambler and Hopkins 1986).

When the stigma is more overt, there is less opportunity to 'pass' as normal (see Chapter 8 for details of coping strategies). In these circumstances, many stigmatized people form their own alternative communities or clubs in which, through meeting people with similar problems, they can feel relatively normal and accepted. Yet, while forming an outside group may help their sense of social isolation, it can further remove and alienate them from so-called normal society. Stigma therefore produces a dilemma for the patient: on the one hand, they can attempt to be part of normal society – yet they will be constantly reminded that they are not 'normal' and risk discovery at any time; on the other hand, they can establish their own 'normal' society of similar outsiders that further alienates them from the bulk of the population.

In part, the response of those stigmatized will be determined by the visibility and obtrusiveness of their stigma. Patients with colostomies (which require the passing of the contents of their colon through a hole in their abdominal wall into a plastic bag worn under their clothing) usually pass as normal, although this might require changes in lifestyle and occasional social embarrassment. Patients with major sensory deficits are more likely to form their own subgroups, but such groups, as pointed out above, can lead to tensions. For example, deaf people can communicate by either lip reading or using hand signs, but because one method tends to dominate, they can be classified either as readers or signers. Readers are obviously better able to cope in a hearing world, yet signers are able, through their more exclusive language, to feel more united as a group (Higgins 1980). Indeed, within the world of the deaf, readers, who can attempt to pass as not deaf, can be stigmatized by signers because they are not committed members of the deaf community.

The dilemma for stigmatized people of choosing whether to be abnormal in a normal world or normal in an abnormal world is also reflected in social and health policy. Disabled children can be educated in a normal school where they will be marked out as abnormal or they can go to a special school where, though their abnormality will not be marked, they will be further removed from normal society. Deaf people can be taught lip reading to enable them to integrate as best they can, or they can be taught sign language to enable them to gain an identity through segregation. The stigmatized can often make the choice themselves, although, because of their organization, commitment and rejection of trying to integrate, it is often those in favour of segregation whose views are heard.

For patients, the management of stigma is a difficult and never-ending task and, while doctors, nurses and other health professionals might not be able to remove the stigma or advise the patients on how best they should run their own lives, there are undoubtedly many occasions when sympathetic counselling and support may be of considerable help (see Chapter 8).

DISABLEMENT

The potentially greater importance of the social reaction to impairment or disability in comparison with the underlying biological deficit was recognized in a well-known model proposed by the World Health Organization (WHO) in 1980 (see Figure 5.1).

The traditional 'medical model' encompasses the specific *physical impairment* and its preceding causes if these were known. Osteoarthritis, short-sightedness and epilepsy are examples of impairment. Physical impairment has two consequences: first it may lead to *functional limitation* and *activity restriction* that together might be labelled as disability; second, through the changes in self-perception and expectation of others (often through stigma), it may create *social handicap*, which in its turn may affect and exacerbate the underlying physical impairment. For most people, the impairment of osteoarthritis only produces disability and, perhaps, some handicap if severe. Short-sightedness produces minimal disability, as it is corrected by spectacles, and little if any handicap (though the popularity of contact lenses suggests that there may be some handicap associ-

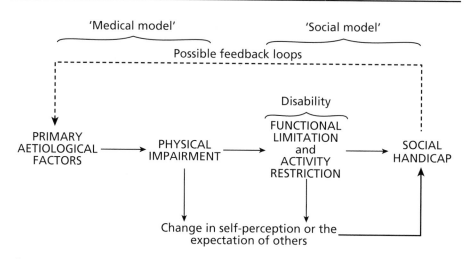

Figure 5.1 World Health Organization: impairment, disability and handicap (after WHO 1980).

ated with spectacle use). Epilepsy in most cases produces minimal disability (if successfully treated), but it still might create significant handicap.

Use of this impairment–disability–handicap model enabled the separate dimensions of the patient's problem to be identified clinically and appropriate management instituted. In addition, it helped clarify the different dimensions of the experience of illness for measurement and research purposes. Despite its utility, however, the classification received criticism from the disability community. In particular, they disliked the idea that they could be handicapped through their disability. Instead, they argued that they were only handicapped to the extent that they lived in a world that placed physical and social barriers to their full participation in everyday life. In other words, the problem was not the disabled person, but the discrimination he or she received from others (Oliver 1996).

Against the idea that disablement was a personal tragedy for the individual that he or she had to manage through adaptation, the new 'social model' claimed it was social oppression that produced problems for disabled people and that the solution was social change. In part, this critique of the WHO classification was a political one. Like any minority group that had its rights restricted by the majority, the disabled community was fighting for recognition and equal rights. Yet, the group did not want to be treated like others, because their needs were very particular. Here again was the dilemma of whether to stress differentness and demand special recognition or to reject differentness and demand to be treated like everyone else. Such policy predicaments cannot easily be resolved, but the WHO has at least tried to address some of these issues in a revised classification that recognizes that disablement is an interaction between the intrinsic features of the individual and that person's social and physical environment. In particular, it replaces 'handicap' with 'participation restrictions' (Bickenbach et al. 1999).

LABELLING AND PSYCHIATRIC DISEASE

Secondary deviance has been used extensively to analyse psychiatry (Ingleby 1981). This is probably for three reasons.

1 Psychiatric diagnosis is less precise than diagnosis in the rest of medicine, with the result that it is easier for the critic to dispute the existence, type or natural history of psychiatric disorders.
2 Unlike most organic diagnoses, psychiatric conditions carry much greater social significance. For centuries madness has been the basis of many and various social theories and practices.
3 The manifestations of mental illness are principally in changed behaviour and, as labelling too may lead to altered behaviour, it may be difficult to distinguish the relative effects of the mental illness itself from the effects of the labelling.

The importance given to the effects of labelling in psychiatry varies from psychiatrist to psychiatrist. Most would now acknowledge the value of labelling in explaining some psychiatric problems; some go as far as to suggest that it can explain all psychiatric morbidity. Three lines of argument can be identified.

PSYCHIATRIC ILLNESS IS A CONSEQUENCE OF THE LABELLING OF PRIMARY DEVIANCE

The main proponent of this view is Thomas Szasz, who argues that mental diseases do not exist in the same way as organic diseases (Szasz 1962). Psychiatric diseases are only metaphors: some people have 'sick' minds in the same way as some economies are 'sick'. The people currently labelled as mentally ill are those whose slightly incongruous behaviour has been labelled and therefore treated by psychiatrists. Thus psychiatrists do not identify 'real' disease, they simply label 'inappropriate' behaviours and call it disease.

Szasz's argument seems to founder on his assumptions about organic disease, in that he believes it to be somehow 'real'. But organic disease only differs from psychiatric disorder in the existence of biological correlates; otherwise, both identify anatomical, physiological or behaviour changes which, it is believed, are socially disadvantageous (see Chapter 14).

Thus, when Szasz claims that psychiatric disease only 'exists' because it is labelled that way, he is not offering a special insight, for this can be argued for all disease. Moreover, such an argument does little to help people who suffer from 'psychiatric phenomena', whatever their status, and it fails to appreciate the way in which social phenomena can have 'real' effects on people's lives.

PSYCHIATRIC ILLNESS IS A CONSEQUENCE OF THE LABELLING OF PRIMARY DEVIANCE AND THE RESULTING SECONDARY DEVIANCE

This view holds that psychiatrists identify a behaviour pattern which, though it may be slightly unusual, is still within the normal range, label it as psychiatric disease (i.e. primary deviance) and, by a process of investigation and treatment, induce the mental illness that was first labelled (i.e. by secondary deviance). The power of this argument stems from two factors:

1 the supposed unsettling impact for someone who is told they are or might be mentally ill: mental illness is still stigmatized and many ex-sufferers try to hide their history;
2 the investigation and treatment environment places the patient in a strange situation in which the 'correct' behaviour is difficult to establish: 'normal' behaviour is clearly abnormal in a mental hospital and, on the other hand, abnormal behaviour merely fulfils the psychiatrist's predictions.

The second point can be illustrated by an experiment conducted in a state hospital in the USA (Rosenhan 1973). The researcher and his co-workers all managed to get themselves admitted by reporting hallucinations the night before. Thereafter, they behaved completely normally – and it took an average of 30 days to get discharged. Behaviour that was normal for the researchers, such as taking notes, was viewed by the staff as bizarre: it was described in the day-book as 'patient engaged in writing behaviour'. The 'patients' who were discharged earliest were those who eventually confessed to having been ill but were now 'feeling better'. Those who continued to profess their normality were kept in longest, as it was believed they were deliberately feigning to get out – clearly pathological behaviour in a mental hospital. (The only people within the hospital to realize the researchers were 'normal' were the other patients!)

Though this study demonstrated the dilemma of appropriate behaviour in a mental hospital, it is uncertain whether it substantiates the labelling perspective. One critic has argued it merely shows the diagnostic ineptitude of the admitting psychiatrists. This is probably the significant point. It is only when early mistakes are made in diagnosis that 'normal' patients are exposed to the potentially unsettling experience of being a patient in a psychiatric setting. Yet it can be argued that because psychiatric diagnostic categories are relatively imprecise, 'mistakes' can be made. Occasionally a mistake is brought to light by the media, but it is impossible without further empirical study to judge the overall impact of this process on the emergence of new psychiatric cases.

PSYCHIATRIC ILLNESS CAN BE EXACERBATED BY LABELLING AND SECONDARY DEVIANCE

The evidence to support this hypothesis comes from patients who have been incarcerated for long periods of time in mental hospitals. They manifest behaviour that is appropriate for the inside of a mental hospital but that is inappropriate for the world outside. This phenomenon of institutionalization denotes the process by which the inmates of large institutions gradually withdraw from normal life and become wholly dependent (Goffman 1961).

Institutionalization is a form of depersonalization induced by 'batch living' whereby patients in large hospitals are processed in groups for feeding, dressing etc. Within this environment, individual autonomy is discouraged as it may interfere with the smooth running of the institution. This means that patients gradually lose their own identity and become increasingly dependent on the hospital and its staff for both major and minor activities. A general apathy pervades their view of life and they have little inclination to want to leave and live independently. Indeed, if discharged, they often have great difficulty adapting to non-hospitalized life, as they cannot manage the most basic decisions of everyday activity (see also Chapter 8).

There is now general awareness of the dangers of prolonged institutionalization, and some of these effects can be combated by minimizing the period of hospitalization and, where hospitalization is necessary, by ensuring a suitable ward environment (Jones and Fowles 1984). Decreasing periods of hospitalization in recent decades (and the concomitant growth of day surgery etc.) has probably significantly reduced the risks of institutionalization in health care, though it remains a potent force elsewhere.

Chapter 6

SOCIAL PATTERNS OF ILLNESS: I

In any population, at any point in time, there will be a variety of different ill-nesses. It is unusual to find any of these illnesses randomly distributed through the population; rather, they tend to form patterns. For example, influenza epidemics usually show temporal patterns, being more common during winter months, and also geographical patterns, as the virus is passed from one person to another through the community. Such patterns are of particular interest because they can:

- often be used to identify the disease or its characteristics,
- suggest causal factors,
- indicate areas of health need that may require more health care provision.

EXPLAINING ILLNESS PATTERNS

The value of looking for patterns of illness is that if the distribution of a disease and a population characteristic (e.g. age, sex, height, blood group, religion etc.) are similar, it suggests that the characteristic is a possible causal or aetiological factor in the disease. For example, to take a hypothetical case, if the distribution of tall people in the community was similar to the distribution of asthma (i.e. asthma was found to be more common in tall people compared with short), the suspicion would emerge that tallness was somehow a contributory cause of asthma. However, an observed correlation such as where there is tallness there is also asthma might also be explained in other ways.

- The causal relationship is, in fact, the other way round: that asthma in men caused them to grow taller. (The importance of knowledge of the temporal order of the variables before imputing causality is discussed in Chapter 4.)
- Something else, say an unknown hormone, causes tallness and asthma, so the two are not causally related at all. (Again, the requirement that the relationship is not spurious in deciding causality is explained in Chapter 4.)
- The observed relationship is an artefact of the measuring process: perhaps the criteria for diagnosing asthma have not been adjusted to take account of the different lung function of tall people so that they seem, mistakenly, to have a higher rate of the disease.

Thus, any similarities between the distribution of illness and population factors need to be treated with caution: on the one hand, patterns of illness can illustrate important aspects of the illness, but on the other, it is all too easy to draw false conclusions. The rest of this chapter and the next therefore describe known relationships between illness and social groupings and, where appropriate, offer evaluations of possible alternative explanations.

HISTORICAL CHANGES

NINETEENTH CENTURY

With the advent of the registration of all deaths in the nineteenth century, it became possible to look for patterns in the distribution of deaths and in their specific causes. Three main configurations of illness stood out in these early studies.

- There was evidence that the death rate varied between different parts of the country. In part, this was a product of the movement of infectious epidemics through the community, but also nineteenth-century epidemiologists noted that mortality rates varied by whether the area was urban or rural. They explained the difference in terms of environmental hazards, particularly those caused by poor sanitation
- With detailed mortality statistics, the nineteenth-century epidemiologist was able to confirm that mortality (and many causes of death) was closely related to age. The infant was particularly at risk; thereafter, mortality declined, before it began its upward climb from middle age.
- In similar fashion, there seemed to be particular risks for males, such as higher infant and occupational mortality as well as an overall shorter life expectancy.

TWENTIETH AND TWENTY-FIRST CENTURIES

The three main nineteenth-century patterns of death described above – namely geography, age and sex – have remained of importance in the twentieth and twenty-first centuries, but the simple story they depicted has been shown to be much more complex.

- The major nineteenth-century patterns of disease distribution – geography, age and sex – which had been viewed solely as manifestations of biological and physical influences within both the body and the environment, have increasingly been linked to psychosocial factors
- Geography, age and sex are not only related to mortality but also to many other aspects of people's lives. This has suggested more complex factors in the aetiology of disease and cause of death. Thus, while mortality was linked to the urban/rural environment, so was poverty; and while the patient's gender predicted his or her life expectancy, it also affected a whole range of other life opportunities. Therefore, by comparing the distribution of mortality with the

distribution of other community characteristics, it became possible to look for other relationships that may have aetiological significance.

* New measures of ill-health, as described in Chapter 3, have enabled more subtle illness patterns to be identified.

When the nineteenth-century epidemiologists examined the relationship of age and sex to mortality, they were subdividing the population in two ways, according to stratified and non-stratified variables. Age is a stratified variable. It might be given in terms of years, or it might be given in terms of age groups or cohorts. Each of these measures represents a scale on which people can be placed, with the implication that one end of the scale has 'more' of the characteristic than the other. Gender, on the other hand, is not stratified, in that maleness and femaleness stand as distinct categories that cannot be ranked. The rest of this chapter examines some non-stratified social patterns that seem to relate to illness; the next chapter deals with stratified patterns.

GEOGRAPHY

As in the nineteenth century, important geographical differences in health persist. Of greatest salience is the disparity in health status between developed and developing parts of the world, but even within industrialized countries there are often significant geographical patterns of illness. For example, the north of England has worse health (in terms of mortality) than the south. Four hypotheses can be advanced to explain this phenomenon.

1 The environmental and occupational hazards are greater in one part of the country (old 'smoke-stack' industries, for example) and these together produce a higher mortality.
2 The finding is an artefact: more working-class people may live in one part of the country and they have greater mortality (see Chapter 7); therefore it is not the region that contributes to higher mortality, but the particular social class/group mix that it contains.
3 There has been a long-term 'drift' of healthier people from one region to another, so affecting the age/sex standardized mortality rate (Bentham 1988; Brimblecombe et al. 2000).
4 Poorer health care facilities in one region compared with another mean that there are more preventable deaths.

It would appear that geographical differences are probably a mixture of all these factors. For example, there is evidence that geographical health differences are not entirely caused by the social mix of the population, as geographical variations exist even within particular social groups. In short, whenever geographical patterning is identified – between countries, between regions, between inner and outer cities etc. – it is likely that there is a number of different factors operating, and the direct effect of physical or biological factors is only one of the explanations.

OCCUPATION

Occupational hazards no doubt still play a part in mortality differences. Also, because last occupation is recorded on the death certificate, it is possible to link various causes of mortality to occupational group and identify those diseases that are found to excess in certain occupations. An example of the sort of picture this can reveal is given in Table 6.1.

Some causes of death are fairly self-explanatory: steel erectors die more frequently from accidental falls, whereas doctors die more frequently from alcohol-induced liver cirrhosis. Others may be artefacts of the measuring process: clerical workers who die from heart disease possibly had the disease before they took up their occupation. Yet others are rather perplexing: why ceramic workers should die more frequently from influenza or maintenance fitters from carcinoma of the colon is unknown. The full list of occupations with their different excess mortalities is a relatively unexplored source of ideas about the aetiology of many diseases.

Many occupations present specific hazards that can determine a particular pattern of mortality and morbidity, but there are other aspects of work that can influence health. A glimpse of these is afforded by the worse health of those without any work (see health effects of unemployment below), but in addition it has been argued that the degree of control exercised by workers over their work can have an important influence on health. Many occupations – medicine being a prime example – involve considerable freedom in determining the day-to-day content of work; other occupations are tightly controlled, offering the worker very little discretion or freedom. It seems that jobs with greater autonomy confer health benefits. For example, in a longitudinal study of civil servants it was found that the degree of job control was a major factor in predicting coronary heart dis-

Table 6.1 Occupational mortality (after OPCS)

Occupation	Disease with excess mortality	Standardized mortality ratio
Ceramic workers	Influenza	780
Steel erectors	Accidental falls	1401
Clerks	Heart disease	143
Electronic engineers	Asthma	561
Doctors	Liver cirrhosis	311
Textile labourers	Duodenal ulcer	367
Maintenance fitters	Cancer of colon	152

All significant: $p < 0.01$.

ease, even after controlling for other risk factors (Marmot et al. 1997). The issue of job control has become such an important feature of occupations that it is now an integral part of thinking about how occupations should be assigned to socio-economic groups (see Chapter 7).

GENDER

Sex differences in mortality have been recorded since the nineteenth century and these are still marked. However, it is now more usual to refer to these as gender differences. A person's sex is simply a biological characteristic; this may have value in examining entirely biological phenomena – such as a disease linked to a sex chromosome – but, as described below, the concept of gender is more useful in the context of the importance of different male and female social roles.

There are two major gender differences in health status in our society that seem to be contradictory.

1 The mortality experience of men is far worse than that of women, women living on average about 5 years longer than men. This suggests that maleness is a major risk factor for ill-health.
2 The morbidity of women seems to be higher than that of men. Measuring morbidity is difficult (see Chapter 3), but, according to at least three measures – namely, surveys of self-reported illness, data on the use of health services and morbidity surveys – women have more illnesses than men.

These findings have led to the claim that 'women get ill but men die'. How is this apparent contradiction to be explained? First, it is important to stress that the explanation is likely to be a social one. There are some diseases that are linked to sex chromosomes and some, such as gynaecological disorders, that are specific to biological sex differences, but most diseases occur in both men and women. Even a possible protective hormonal balance for women is challenged by the continuation of preferential survival after the menopause. In addition, there is cross-cultural evidence of different patterns of disease between the sexes (in which it is the men who seem to get more illnesses and women who have shorter life expectancy) that also challenges the view that their diseases are biologically fixed. So what are the possible explanations for the higher illness rate in women and higher mortality rate in men?

One possibility is that the types of illnesses suffered by men and women are different. Diseases that cause death, such as heart disease, are different from the diseases that cause non-fatal illnesses, such as most skin diseases; men may have more of the former and women more of the latter.

It has been argued that the diseases that cause death, in particular heart disease and cancer, are closely linked with male lifestyle in our society. Men seem to be more competitive and aggressive: they are therefore more likely to indulge in health-harming activities – smoking, alcohol, bad diet etc. – as a coping response, and this, combined with the direct effect of these stressors, leads to a higher incidence of fatal diseases (Waldron 1976). However, these differences in lifestyle seem to be changing – for example smoking rates in men and women are becoming similar – so that the gap in mortality rates is beginning to narrow, particularly for older middle-aged adults, while suicides and AIDS seem to be widening the gap for younger people (Waldron 1993).

The second explanation is that it is differential access to health care that may explain at least some of the mortality differences, that is, because women are higher users of health care, they benefit from medical diagnosis and treatments. This explanation assumes that medical intervention can make a major contribution to extending life expectancy, and there is little evidence to support such a massive effect; indeed, McKeown (1979) argued that medicine overall had had only a marginal effect on longevity. Moreover, when access to 'life-saving' treatments such as cardiac surgery is compared, the picture often, paradoxically, seems to favour men (Dong et al. 1998).

The third explanation for male/female differences in illness is that of women's social position. Women have different sorts of stressors from men that may well lead to higher illness rates. Women's traditional role is more passive and dependent, and their subsidiary social status often engenders low self-esteem. Taken together, these aspects of women's social status may produce many minor illnesses, particularly mental health problems. If women have the same occupational and social environments as men – which can be examined by comparing men and women in similar jobs and circumstances – their rate of minor psychiatric disturbance is no worse than that of men (Jenkins 1985; Emslie et al. 1999).

However, it is not simply a question of comparing paid jobs if domestic responsibilities remain a major part of a woman's role. Women's higher morbidity risk has been shown to be based on less involvement in paid work, greater felt stress and unhappiness, and stronger feelings of vulnerability to illness (Verbrugge 1989). Another study found that women in paid employment do seem to have better health, but only if over 40 years of age or without children; young mothers with full-time work have worse health unless they have access to adequate resources to help cope with their multiple roles (Arber et al. 1985). In summary, whereas in general paid work is protective of women's health, domestic roles and responsibilities can easily override this positive influence. It means that if a man and woman both experience the same adverse life event, it will be largely the woman's domestic burden that will determine her greater vulnerability (Nazroo et al. 1998).

The fourth explanation for differences in illness rates between men and women is that it is an artefact of differential reporting (and the associated increase in help-seeking behaviour). According to this perception-reporting hypothesis, women are more likely to perceive, recall and report symptoms than men (Verbrugge 1985). For example, in a group of patients with mild hypertension, women were twice as likely to report their health as poor and reported many more symptoms than men – though these differences largely disappeared when account was taken of their psychological state (Anson et al. 1993). Yet establishing whether or not a person is faithfully reporting his or her 'real' health status is a difficult task, and there are other studies that find no gender differences in illness reporting (Macintyre et al. 1999).

Overall, it would appear that the reasons for differences in health status between men and women revolve around their social positions: men's social roles produce mortality hazards, whereas a woman's social role not only makes her vulnerable to more illnesses but also affects her perceptions of those illnesses. In this sense, it is less gender per se that determines illness than the particular social circumstances that gender implies in contemporary society. As these circumstances change – for women and for men – the gender relationship to health is also likely to change.

ETHNICITY

Until the mid-1960s, it was common to classify groups of people by their racial characteristics. In the main, this meant skin colour, but the assumption was that there were important biological differences between these racial groups. A century later, these biological differences look a lot less important than they did – and it is realized that skin colour is often a poor predictor of racial origins. Certainly there are some genetic diseases, the haemoglobinopathies for example, that cluster by racial origin, but most of the differences between people from different parts of the world seem to be based on culture rather than biology, as disease patterns seem to change in immigrants who adopt the culture of their host country.

As race has declined in value as a system of classification, the idea of ethnicity has emerged to take its place. Ethnicity refers to a social group that is held together by a common culture, perhaps built around language, history or religion. Unlike race, ethnicity is based on people's identification with a particular social group, in particular individual self-assessment of which social group they belong to – which might bear little relationship to their apparent skin colour.

Information on a person's ethnicity is collected in the decennial census but is less commonly collected during routine health care. There is disagreement about the best classification system to use, but also there is sensitivity about asking for ethnicity data given the history of racism. The study of ethnic differences in health is therefore less well developed than the work on, say, gender or social class. Nevertheless, from the limited ethnic monitoring carried out, a number of health differences have been reported among ethnic groups in the population, for example higher rates of ischaemic heart disease amongst Asians, greater prevalence of strokes and hypertension among those of Afro-Caribbean descent. So how are these to be explained?

BIOLOGICAL DIFFERENCES

As noted above, there are some health problems that have a genetic basis and some of these are clustered by ethnic group. However, for many of these differences, the effect of culture is much greater. For Japanese women living in Japan, for example, breast cancer is a rare event, but when they migrate to the USA and adopt American diets, lifestyles etc., their cancer rate increases to equal that of women in their host country. Certainly there might be a breast cancer gene operating for many of these women, but it seems to be environmental factors that allow it expression.

If biological factors have any important role, it may be in the process of migration, as healthier than average individuals 'select' themselves for movement to another country (Marmot et al. 1984). This means that 'healthier' genes are being selectively favoured in the migration process. In addition, of course, the social ties that immigrants bring and maintain in their host country may have an influence on their patterns of illness – though this reflects the influence of culture rather than biology (Marmot and Syme 1976).

ARTEFACT EXPLANATIONS

Almost by definition, different ethnic groups have different lifestyles: so is it the ethnic group or the particular lifestyle that produces observable health differences? Put another way, does the fact that many British Asian communities are strongly working class in terms of their occupations account for their worse health? Does knowing their ethnicity add anything?

The answer is: much less than it seemed from the raw differences, in that allowing for the socio-economic position of ethnic minorities explains much of the health differential (Davey Smith 2000). For example, people from the Indian subcontinent in Britain report poorer self-rated health than the white community. Yet if the figures are adjusted to take account of the social class, local area deprivation and standard of living, most of the differences disappear (Chandola 2001). It is also possible that some of the unexplained differences can be understood in terms of limitations in the measurement processes: perhaps a better (and more appropriate for ethnic minorities) measure of socio-economic position would explain even more. This therefore raises the question: what is an ethnic group? Is it simply the clustering of socio-economic and lifestyle factors, a shorthand way of referring to a particular health risk configuration? Or is it something more?

THE MINORITY EXPERIENCE

What many ethnic groups have in common is their minority status. Being a black African in Africa is very different from being a black African in a predominantly white British society, all other things being equal. This points to a component of being an ethnic minority that cannot be accounted for in terms of socio-economic status and lifestyle factors. Ethnicity provides both a social structure and an identity (Smaje 1996; Nazroo 1998). Being a member of an ethnic minority may confer health advantages, particularly through feelings of social support and solidarity within that community (see Chapter 4), but, equally, the minority experience is also so often one of prejudice and stigma. For example, the higher rates of mental disorder reported in the black community may be a response to a lifetime of discrimination in all its forms, but also it is possible that some behaviour patterns more frequently found in certain ethnic cultures may become labelled as psychiatric illness (Littlewood and Lipsedge 1981).

UNEMPLOYMENT

Economic retrenchment that occurs periodically in Western countries produces unemployment and there is evidence that those who are unemployed have higher rates of mortality and illness.

The effects of unemployment can be divided into psychological and material. For a minority, unemployment will be welcomed. They may have sufficient income from redundancy money, pension and state benefits etc. and be released from what might be a hazardous work environment. In addition, leaving certain forms of work behind may reduce stress and give an opportunity to engage in valued activities. In such cases it might be expected that unemployment would produce beneficial effects on health.

For the vast majority, however, unemployment forms a major life crisis. There is a fall in income that will affect the material resources available to the unemployed and their family. There are also major psychological changes: the unemployed person suffers loss of role and way of life; there is a loss of social contacts that were maintained through work; there is loss of self-esteem; and there is anxiety about the future and feelings of rejection. Many of these harmful health effects may extend to the families of the unemployed.

Taken together, these various observations about the experience of unemployment would suggest that it is likely that unemployed people would experience more illness. In fact, the evidence from mortality figures and from morbidity surveys does support this inference (Moser et al. 1987; Arber 1987). Yet, before the observed correlation between illness and unemployment can be taken as evidence that unemployment *causes* illness, it is necessary to consider two alternative explanations.

A SPURIOUS RELATIONSHIP

It is possible that it is not unemployment alone that is causing ill-health, but another, third, variable acting with it. For example, it is known that working-class men are more likely to be unemployed at any point in time compared with middle-class men and, probably for independent reasons (see Chapter 7), working-class men are likely to have more illnesses and higher mortality than middle-class men. Therefore, in any sample of unemployed men there is likely to be a higher proportion of working-class men who are more likely to be ill. Thus a correlation might be found between unemployment and ill-health, but it is not a causal one.

This explanation can be examined more closely by controlling for the third variable, in this case social class. This is done by looking at illness patterns within social class groups. If illness is linked to unemployment rather than social class, holding social class steady by, say, looking at all men in Social Class V and comparing those who are employed and unemployed, will mean that any differences must be independent of social class. When this calculation is carried out, there is still a 20–30 per cent excess mortality in the unemployed (Moser et al. 1984).

An investigation of parasuicide (attempted suicide) in Edinburgh examined another variable in the link between unemployment and ill-health (Platt and Kreitman 1984). Looking at small areas of the city, the researchers discovered a high correlation between unemployment and parasuicide. After controlling for social class (as described above), this correlation was reduced but was still significant: in other words, there was a still a strong link between the experience of unemployment and attempted suicide. However, after controlling for yet another variable, namely poverty, the relationship between unemployment and parasuicide disappeared. This suggested that poverty had a more important role to play in the production of parasuicide than unemployment, though poverty and unemployment are clearly linked.

TEMPORAL ORDERING

It is possible that there is a causal link between unemployment and ill-health but that the relationship is the reverse temporal order. In other words, ill-health tends to cause unemployment.

All unemployed men do not become ill; it is only a greater tendency to be ill that shows up in the figures. However, perhaps this observed correlation between unemployment and ill-health is caused by the greater likelihood of ill people being made unemployed. If a business is going to make, say, 10 per cent of its workforce redundant, it is probably more likely to offer redundancy to those workers whose health record is in some way impaired. In effect, there would be a selection factor in the creation of unemployment that would tend to push the ill members of the population into the unemployed group.

To test for this explanation, it is necessary to use longitudinal studies that track groups of patients over time. Ideally, one would start with a healthy work force and examine people's illness and unemployment careers thereafter. One study looked at the health records of school leavers and followed them for several years, examining their employment record and their health changes (Banks and Jackson 1982). It was found that those school leavers who became unemployed did seem to experience more minor psychiatric disease, even allowing for their original health status. However, an Australian investigation that followed 8000 young people through their experiences in the job market noted the importance of job satisfaction for mental health (Graetz 1993). There was a decline in the mental health of those who went into jobs that were dissatisfying; equally, those who resigned from jobs in which they had found no satisfaction reported an improvement in their mental health. The study confirmed that employment and job satisfaction interacted, with the dissatisfied employed having worse mental health than the unemployed.

Another study to look at the effect of unemployment on health involved examining the mortality of men over a 10-year period, starting with a group of men in 1971 who were either in employment or unemployed and seeking work (Moser et al. 1984). Permanently unemployed people who were chronically sick were excluded from the study. The results showed that the group of men seeking work in 1971 had particularly high mortality rates in the following decade from cancers, accidents, poisoning and violence. The other interesting finding in the study was that the wives of unemployed men also had relatively high mortality rates, suggesting a direct effect of unemployment rather than a selection effect.

Again, it is possible to explain the findings of this study with reference to other variables. The study itself allowed for the effect of social class so as to show that the impact of unemployment was independent of social standing. However, it is still possible that those men seeking work in 1971 were in some way less healthy than their working colleagues, and this could explain their increased mortality. It is also already known that mortality between spouses is linked: the death of one spouse is more likely to be followed by the death of the other. Therefore, the higher mortality rates amongst the wives of unemployed men may also be accounted for by this other intra-family dynamic factor, rather than by unemployment itself.

The studies linking unemployment and ill-health demonstrate some of the considerable difficulties in disentangling causal relationships in the social sciences. As things stands, it is probably reasonable to conclude that the evidence points to a causal link between unemployment and ill-health; indeed it would appear that even the experience of a short period of unemployment seems to reduce people's 'health capital' and make them susceptible to illnesses later in their lives (Wadsworth et al. 1999).

Chapter 7

SOCIAL PATTERNS OF ILLNESS: II

AGE

As nineteenth-century epidemiologists observed, overall mortality is closely related to age. It is not, however, a simple linear relationship, but rather a lopsided U-curve. This is because mortality is still, despite major improvements since the nineteenth century, relatively high in infants under 1 year old; mortality then declines rapidly, before picking up again in middle age and rising steeply in the elderly. In keeping with this distribution of all deaths, many specific causes of death are similarly closely related to increasing age. For example, cancer and heart disease, the major causes of death in the Western world, are much more common in the elderly than in the young. On the other hand, some diseases stand out as being only found in younger age groups: certain leukaemias, for example, are mostly found in childhood.

Just as there is a clear relationship between the pattern of mortality and age, there is similar supportive evidence to relate morbidity to age. First, the elderly report more illnesses; second, in studies of the prevalence of chronic illness, using activities of daily living as a measure, most of the illness is concentrated among the elderly; and third, from caseload data it is known that they go more frequently to the doctor.

It is customary to presume that the relationship between chronological age and illness is a product of biological decline associated with the ageing process. However, it is possible to argue that ageing is also a socio-cultural process, and some of the health problems of older people relate to the social process of ageing rather than to biological involution. Support for this argument can be obtained from three sources.

1 The improvements in overall life expectancy over the last century or so suggest that many deaths are not as biologically inevitable as was once believed. It is now known that one of the prime determinants of infant mortality is not the fixed biological nature of the infant, but rather its environment. Improvements in standard of living, such as have occurred since the nineteenth century, have also reduced infant mortality (McKeown 1979).

Similarly, many of the diseases of ageing have been shown to have environmental/social causes. It has been calculated that up to 80 per cent of all cancers are environmentally determined. Amongst other things, smoking, diet and exercise have all been implicated in coronary heart disease, which is itself highly correlated with age. All of these factors suggest that the biological decline of the body is not as fixed as once assumed, and it would appear that social factors play a part in the illnesses of ageing as much as biological factors. Indeed, there is a model of human ageing that predicts that the constantly improving health of the population will result in the 'compression of morbidity', in which illness is reduced to the few years at the end of the 'natural' life span of about 85 years (Fries 1980). This may already be happening, though it is probably restricted to those who are more highly educated (Crimmins and Saito 2001).

2 There is evidence that many of the so-called biological changes with ageing are in fact culturally specific. In other words, the biological changes known to accompany ageing in modern Western societies are not found elsewhere. For example, blood pressure is known to increase with age – in some people excessively so, producing hypertension – but in other societies there is no increase with age (Henry and Cassel 1969). It is therefore possible that many of the changes that have been accepted as inevitable are in fact the product of environmental conditions.

3 The final piece of the jigsaw that suggests ageing has a social component as well as a biological one is the specific way older people are treated. Several years ago there was a theory that elderly people gradually disengage from social life. This was believed to be due to biological changes that prevented them from participating fully in usual activities, and because of their desire to leave the hurry and bustle of everyday life. In retrospect, this theory is now seen to be limited, and it is possible that many old people were 'disengaged' whether they wanted to be or not. As labelling theory suggests (see Chapter 5), treating old people as if they were disengaging is likely to produce the very phenomenon that it predicts. From what is now known of the importance of labelling and social support, this forcible disengagement might have had damaging health effects. It would therefore appear that it is not only the actual biological decline of ageing that determines illness patterns, but also the presumed biological decline, which then affects the social reaction to and treatment of old people and, in its turn, their illnesses.

SOCIAL CLASS

In the nineteenth century it was observed that certain causes of mortality seemed to be linked to various occupations and occupational groups. In part, this was a result of specific work hazards; but occupation was also linked to way of life, which might, in turn, be related to illness. For example, certain occupations were far better paid than others, meaning that the person concerned could expect better housing, nutrition and so on.

CLASSIFICATION

In an attempt to encapsulate these wider aspects of occupations, early in the twentieth century the British Registrar-General devised a system of classifying occupations into eight different groups, or social classes, that would convey something of their social standing and skills. The Registrar-General then showed that there was a close relationship between each social class and its overall infant mortality rate (deaths of children under the age of 1 year with a denominator of total live births in the period). In short, these groupings of occupations were powerfully predictive of the health risk to infants born into these classes; and these risks to infants did not seem to be directly linked to the specific work hazards of particular occupations. The Registrar-General later reduced the social classes from eight to five groups (see Table 7.1).

Other systems of social stratification exist in other countries and for other purposes – the A to E system used to describe consumers in market research, the division into a larger number of socio-economic groups and, a new one in Britain, the National Statistics Socio-Economic Classification (NS-SEC: see below) – but all follow a similar pattern. In some analyses the different social-class groups are aggregated to form two broad divisions, non-manual and manual; these are often referred to as middle and working class, or white-collar and blue-collar workers.

In principle, people are assigned to a social class on the basis of their occupation; in practice, it is not quite so simple. There are many people without an occupation, so that it is difficult to classify them. One general rule for such people is to use their male head of household: this means that children can be classified by their father's occupation, as can wives who are not in the labour market. However, the retired, the unemployed, single women and 'working wives' still pose difficulties – as do some occupational groups that do not fall within the classification system, such as students and the armed forces. Sometimes such people are simply omitted from the analysis; alternatively, other ways can be found of classifying them: retired and unemployed can be assigned according to their last

Table 7.1 Social classes

Middle or non-manual class	
Social class I	Professional
Social class II	Employers and managers
Social class III (non-manual)	Intermediate and junior non-manual
Working or manual class	
Social class III (manual)	Skilled manual and own account non-professional
Social class IV	Semi-skilled manual and personal services
Social class V	Unskilled manual

occupation; single women can be classified according to their own occupation and working women to their husbands' social classes.

The practice of assigning women to their husbands' social classes, even when the majority have their own jobs that could be used as the basis of classification, has come in for severe criticism. Why should women be classified according to their husbands' occupations, rather than their own, in some Victorian display of familial male supremacy? The arguments against this criticism are:

- classifying women according to their own occupation would still leave those not in the labour market to be classified by their husbands' occupations;
- women in the work force tend not to be spread around such a range of jobs as men, with the result that a policy of classifying them according to their own occupations would lose some of the discriminatory power of following male occupation patterns;
- at the end of the day, it is the power of social class to explain illness that counts, and the occupation of the male head of household is usually a better predictor of illness than the woman's own job.

Part of the problem is in deciding whether social class is a property of an individual or a household, and this again relates to which has the greater explanatory power. One solution to these difficulties is to change the classification system to make it easier to accommodate these other groups in the population, and various attempts have been made to develop a new classification that will be easier to operate. Levels of education and of income both correlate with health status but pose their own problems of measurement. Level of education needs to accommodate the fact that in earlier decades the school-leaving age was lower and fewer people proceeded to tertiary education; educational attainment differences cannot therefore be easily compared across different age groups. Income seems a good predictor, but stipulating whether the figure should be before or after tax, with or without bonuses and pension contributions etc. makes it difficult to define, quite apart from the sensitivity felt by many people about revealing their exact earnings in a survey.

Although social class is a good predictor of health (and much else), there is debate about what being in a certain social class actually means. What is being measured when someone is assigned to a social grouping on the basis of his or her occupation? Sometimes it seemed to be measuring skill levels or expertise, at other times, a sort of general standing in the community. In an attempt to produce a more meaningful classification, the Office of National Statistics in Britain introduced the National Statistics Socio-Economic Classification, which attempts to place people into groups on the basis of the autonomy they exercise over the content of their work. The logic for selecting control over work as an underlying theme can be seen in the well-established relationship between autonomy and heart disease (see Chapter 6). The new classification broadly follows the previous one because, by and large, people in managerial and professional occupations exercise more control over their work than employees in routine occupations. Even so, ironically, despite its new conceptual coherence, it may not be as powerful as the old classification in terms of predicting ill-health (Chandola 2000).

DIFFERENCES

Despite the difficulties of measuring social class, there is now sufficient accumulated evidence to show that social stratification has an important relationship to health and illness.

- Mortality in all age groups is known to vary by social class. Stillbirths, perinatal mortality (stillbirths plus deaths in the first week of life), infant mortality, childhood mortality and adult mortality in all age cohorts are known to be greater in lower socio-economic groups than in higher ones, with a gradient between the two.
- The more limited evidence that exists for the distribution of morbidity throughout the community (see Chapter 3) indicates that social class is closely linked to this measure of illness. Thus, for example, surveys that have explored self-reported morbidity, both acute and chronic, suggest more illness in lower social classes compared with higher, with the familiar gradient between the two (Blaxter 1990).
- Subjective measures of health status suggest worse health for those lower down the social-class scale. For example, a social-class profile established using the Nottingham Health Profile found that for energy, pain, emotional reactions, sleep and physical mobility there was a clear class gradient, with those lower on the social-class scale having the worst health (Hunt et al. 1986).

EXPLANATIONS

Social-class differences in health have been of particular interest to sociologists for two reasons.

1 Many sociologists believe that the social-class divisions of modern Western societies are fundamental to understanding how they both change and maintain their stability. The links with health are therefore just one more facet of a much larger explanatory framework.
2 Linked to the above, social class is associated with many other features of modern society. Social class relates to income, housing, education, leisure activities, diet etc., so that each of these may also be linked with illness.

Various explanations have been advanced for the observed close association between health and social class.

Material explanations

One of the remarkable features of social-class stratification is how it relates to many other aspects of life, such as income, education, housing etc. This means that working-class people have poorer access overall to resources than middle-class people, and this led to a claim that this relative material deprivation is the major factor in producing higher morbidity and mortality in working-class groups.

This explanation certainly has appeal. It was, in fact, the major explanation accepted by the Black Report, a working party set up to look at social-class inequalities in the context of the National Health Service in Britain (Townsend and Davidson 1982). Because the relationship between social class, health and material resources is so close and consistent, it does provide a very strong case that these material circumstances are implicated in the causation of illness. Furthermore, evidence from the nineteenth century (discussed in Chapter 6) supports the idea that it is relative standard of living that is the major determinant of health status. If this is correct, material deprivation could be corrected by directing additional resources towards those families in need (Townsend et al. 1988).

Nevertheless, although the association between social class and illness is very close, and the general argument seems so reasonable, critics can point to the lack of known mechanisms linking material deprivation to ill-health. Diet, for example, and other environmental factors that might be influenced by poor resources have been suggested to be of aetiological significance, but the relationship between specific dietary habits and disease is not at all clear cut. Dietary items such as cholesterol and vegetables may be important, but their exact role in the causation of many diseases remains confused. The very fact that there is such a debate about the effects of these specific dietary factors also suggests that their influence, if shown, will not be large enough to explain the size of social-class variation.

In the nineteenth century, the association between the poor housing of the working class and illness was probably mainly brought about by lack of running water and unhygienic conditions. Today, it is more likely to be relative overcrowding, dampness, and coldness in winter, but it is difficult to correlate high overall mortality with each of these factors. Specific cases can be pointed to, such as hypothermia amongst old people, or asthma and chest infections in children, but on their own these are insufficient to explain the very large differences in morbidity and mortality between the social classes.

Nevertheless, housing may still be important because in recent years it has been suggested that housing tenure (in particular whether a person owns his or her own house, often with a mortgage, or rents) may give a better prediction of health status (Morgan 1983) or health behaviours (Pill et al. 1993), and it is relatively easily measured. It has been found, for example, that owner-occupiers are more likely to have better health than those in rented accommodation. Housing tenure, of course, cuts across social class: middle-class people tend to be owner-occupiers, but there are people with Social Class I jobs who live in rented accommodation and people with Social Class V jobs who own their own houses. However, in these instances, the type of housing tenure seems more important than social class in predicting health status. This may have something to do with the quality of the housing, but, equally, housing tenure may also reflect other attributes of the person such as income, job security, independence etc., which in their turn may be the real determinants of health.

In summary, there are some specific diseases that can be precisely related to working-class material deprivation. Accidents in childhood, for example, both in the home and outside, probably relate to poor domestic facilities and to lack of safe playing areas outside the home. However, taken together, all these specific links between material circumstance and illness do not add up to an adequate explanation for the large differences between social classes.

A much more powerful explanation of illness is afforded by specific habits, such as cigarette smoking. At first sight, smoking is not a measure of deprivation but of relative prosperity, given that the habit is quite costly. Nevertheless, it has been argued that smoking is, in fact, a response to material deprivation. A working-class family, without the material resources that may be commonplace for a middle-class family, may find that smoking is a means of coping with their lives (Graham 1987). In this sense, smoking is a consequence of material deprivation, and the high morbidity and mortality that can be associated with it support the notion that it is material deprivation that produces illness, albeit indirectly. Alternatively, the smoking evidence can be used to argue that it is not material deprivation but beliefs and customs of the social-class group that produce illness.

Cultural explanations

It is known that different societies, even at the same stage of economic development, have different patterns of disease. For example, the major cause of death amongst men in the USA is heart disease, whereas in Japan it is stroke (cerebrovascular accident). When Japanese men emigrate to the USA, however, and become acculturated to that society, their mortality pattern changes, as they die more frequently from coronary heart disease (Marmot et al. 1975). This phenomenon cannot be explained in terms of material deprivation, as there is little difference in standard of living between Japan and the USA. The only alternative is that it is something to do with the way of life in the two countries that contributes to the particular disease patterns to be found. It may be nutrition, health behaviours or family dynamics, but whatever it is, it is rooted in the particular cultural milieu in which people find themselves.

This argument can be applied to social-class differences in health. In many ways, the different lifestyles of the middle and working classes constitute different cultures. They have different habits, read different newspapers, watch different television programmes, pursue different leisure activities, have different outlooks on life and so on. This can be seen, for example, in poor working-class support for illness prevention programmes.

Yet even if some class differences in health can be explained by different class cultures, there is probably still a close relationship with material deprivation. The culture itself may be a response to long-term material deprivation and, further, the culture may in various ways hinder material improvement. One theory of the 1960s was that as living standards for working-class people improved, they would start to embrace a middle-class way of life. A major study of the relatively affluent workers in a car plant showed that, despite their increased income, working-class culture still prevailed: there may be change, but it is likely to occur over a long period of time.

Another factor in the relationship between cultural explanations of ill-health and material deprivation is the observation that higher mortality is found in those

Western countries that have the widest range of income distribution (Wilkinson 1990, 1996), though there continues to be debate about this observation (Mackenbach 2002). Individuals may not be overtly aware of the range of income distribution, but somehow it may affect their health. A link with the idea of social capital (see Chapter 4) has been suggested as a possible mechanism – and here again it seems to be inequality (as measured by incomes) that contributes to the health status of a population. Thus, economic growth may not lead to optimum health gain if major social inequalities persist.

If the material explanation is correct, then there is a direct policy implication: material deprivation can be corrected by targeting of new resources. However, if a cultural explanation is correct, then the policy implications are not so clear. First, it is probably much more difficult to change a cultural pattern. For example, campaigns to get working-class people to stop smoking have been largely unsuccessful. Second, there is an ethical issue in trying to change aspects of culture. If, for example, a working-class man smokes because he finds pleasure in the activity and he is less concerned about the long-term consequences, do middle-class health professionals have a right to tell him that his values are mistaken and that he should substitute deferred gratification for immediate? There is evidence that cigarette smoking is an integral component of the lifestyle of many working-class people; is it morally right to try to change this for a middle-class value?

Artefact explanations

The central feature of the artefact explanation is that the observed and supposedly causal relationship between social class and illness is spurious: it is not that social class causes illness, but that in some way illness causes the person to belong to a particular social class (Bloor et al. 1987). Three variants of this position can be identified.

Drift and social class The relationship between social class and illness is determined by identifying people's occupations, which places them in a social class, and relating this class position with their health status. But perhaps it is not occupation/social class that influences illness, but illness that influences social class. For example, a Social Class I lawyer with schizophrenia may be unable to continue in his or her chosen occupation and eventually takes a relatively unskilled job. This phenomenon may account for at least some of the excess numbers of Social Class V people with schizophrenia. The argument might also apply to other diseases, such as heart and respiratory diseases, which might cause people to change their occupation. It is therefore possible that the social-class variation in illness is a product of occupational changes following the advent of illness, rather than the other way round.

The drift downward (or upward mobility) hypothesis is limited by the lack of occupational mobility in the retired, children and married women, and even for those in employment it may be more the accumulation of disadvantage that explains the effects of selection (Blane et al. 1993). Even so, for certain diseases, occupational 'drift' is a component of the explanation of social-class variation, though for other diseases there may be some drift towards middle-class office jobs

and away from manual jobs. A major longitudinal study that examined the prevalence of chronic ill-health in men over a 20-year period tried to disentangle these
effects by examining the health status of those who moved between social classes
(Bartley and Plewis 1997). It was found that those who were upwardly mobile
tended to have better health than those in the class they were leaving but worse
health than those in the class they were joining, and vice versa for those who were
downwardly mobile. In effect, social mobility acted to constrain rather than
increase class differences for these illnesses.

Infant mortality and social class Is it possible that the observed relationship
between social class and illness is simply a product of the way that social class
itself is measured? This hypothesis arose out of the process through which social
class was originally derived by the Registrar-General at the beginning of the twentieth century. His purpose was to show that infant mortality was related to social
class. To this end, he classified occupations into eight broad groupings and then
showed that the higher the grouping the lower the infant mortality rate. But how
did he assign occupations to these eight different categories?

The assignment could not have been an entirely arbitrary procedure, otherwise
he would have found no relationship with infant mortality. It is therefore possible that he already knew the infant mortality rate of each occupational group, and
used this as the basis of assignment; in other words, he might have assigned occupations with a high infant mortality rate to a low social class and vice versa. His
finding that social class was related to infant mortality would then be a circular
argument: yes, there was a relationship between the two, but only because social
class had been defined in terms of infant mortality (Jones and Cameron 1984).

It is doubtful that the Registrar-General deliberately 'fixed' his findings, but
neither is it clear what he actually did. He may, as he suggested himself, have
assigned occupations on the basis of social standing, which would have embraced
those crucial aspects of social class such as housing, behaviour, education, wealth
etc., which were then, as now, believed to have a powerful influence on infant
mortality. The suspicion remains, however, that there is something slightly circular about the method of constructing his occupational groupings.

The suspicion of circularity in the relationship between social class and health
is reinforced by the knowledge that occupations are regularly reassigned between
social classes. Every 10 years, the distribution of occupations in their social
classes was reassessed, and sometimes occupations were moved. This was justified
on the grounds that the work of specific occupations can change with new technology and the acquisition of new skills. On these grounds, an occupation that
might have been decidedly unskilled 50 years ago could now be seen as skilled,
and vice versa. It was therefore important that this change was recognized in the
social-class classification. But how much change in any occupation's task was
needed to justify reassignment? No doubt it was the whole panoply of social-class
indicators, such as income, education, housing etc., that helped determine this;
but also, perhaps, it was the occupation's infant mortality rate and/or health status (which is associated with these other attributes of social class) that affected

reassignment, even if indirectly. In this way, the continuing social-class differential in mortality this century could be an artefact of constant re-classifications: whenever an occupation improved its mortality rate, it was simply moved up the scale to a new class, leaving the old class with a residuum of high-risk occupations.

Although this explanation may have appeal for conspiracy theorists, social-class membership is not simply determined by health status. As pointed out above, social class also correlates highly with many other facets of living. In this way, it appears a more meaningful category than would have been produced by some arbitrary procedures. Nevertheless, it is still possible that a certain amount of the observed gradient between social classes has been maintained by the regular reassignment of some occupations. This means that mortality data by social class from one decade are not directly comparable with mortality data by social class from another; some studies have tried to correct for this reassignment factor, but they cannot correct for the fact that the mix of occupations in a social class changes, as does the nature of occupations themselves.

If assignment of occupations was based on health status, some degree of homogeneity might be expected between the social classes. However, what is remarkable is the great diversity of health status, even within a social class. In other words, the construction of social classes may be concealing differences rather than amplifying them. This view is supported by a study of different grades of civil servants that showed the gradient between high and low to be considerably greater than their nominal class position would indicate (Rose and Marmot 1981).

Social class and coronary heart disease The final artefactual explanation relates not to overall mortality and morbidity rates but to specific causes. It is now known that Social Classes IV and V have a higher mortality from coronary heart disease than Social Classes I and II. Forty years ago, however, the relationship was the other way round. It is now suggested that the inverse relationship in the past was an artefact of the measuring process. This could have come about for two reasons.

1 Cause of death is established by clinicians and pathologists: there are, no doubt, fashions in diagnosis and it is possible that in the inter-war years the relatively newly fashionable label of coronary heart disease was diagnosed more frequently in middle-class than in working-class people.

   In the inter-war years, many people received a diagnosis of myocardial degeneration; this diagnosis is now not acceptable and, in retrospect, many of these deaths may well have been cases of coronary heart disease. It is possible, therefore, that if diagnostic fashions are themselves class related, this may produce artificial excesses or shortages of particular illnesses in different social groups.

2 The other reason for a falsely high rate of deaths from coronary heart disease in middle-class men relates to the numerators and denominators used in the calculation. To determine a rate of coronary heart disease deaths, the number

of deaths from the disease in a particular group must be known, as well as the numbers at risk. Thus, the social-class death rate for coronary heart disease involves dividing the numerator of number of deaths in a particular class by the denominator, which would be the total numbers in that social class in the population. (These figures would usually also be standardized to allow for age and sex variations between social classes.)

The denominator is determined from census data, which are produced every 10 years. The census asks a question about occupation that enables numbers in each social class (and therefore 'at risk') to be determined. The numerator is obtained from death certificates that record from the relatives' report the deceased's last occupation. Thus error can creep in from using a denominator that is out of date or a numerator that is inaccurate.

The existence of an apparent excess number of deaths from coronary heart disease among middle-class men led to the 1960s belief in diseases of affluence: that the ravages of disease that had so afflicted the poor in the nineteenth century were now turning their attention to the rich. In retrospect, this argument is now thought to be mistaken, because it is unlikely that middle-class people during this period did have excessive mortality from coronary heart disease. Moreover, it is also mistaken to argue that modern society is characterized by diseases of affluence. Certainly there are diseases brought about by over-consumption, alcoholism being one, but, by and large, the illnesses in our community seem to be associated, as in the nineteenth century, with deprivation in its widest sense.

THE LIFE COURSE

The extensive literature on social class has tended to focus on comparisons between groups in terms of their immediate illnesses and deaths. In recent years, a new form of analysis has emerged that tries to combine two aspects of illness patterning, social class and age, in the 'life course' (van de Meehn et al. 1998). This perspective recognizes that inequality is not a momentary characteristic of someone's life, but is probably the product of a lifetime of deprivation. Thus, the seeds of later illnesses – and inequalities – are often laid down in childhood and in early adult life. It is only by studying these temporal changes that patterns of later inequality can be placed in context and some of its precursors better understood. For example, if *in utero* nutrition is a strong predictor of illness in later life (Barker 1992), does not this indicate the need to intervene preventively as well as at the time the illness appears?

Chapter 8

COPING WITH ILLNESS

People cope with illness in a variety of different ways and in so doing call upon a range of resources. Acute illness tends to be the least difficult to manage, simply because it is by definition a temporary situation. Chronic illness, on the other hand, usually requires more fundamental readjustments on behalf of both patients and their immediate carers. These various coping strategies can, in their turn, help ameliorate the impact of the illness or, in certain circumstances, worsen the situation.

MANAGING LABELS

One response to a diagnostic label is behaviour change (secondary deviance); this consequence of labelling is discussed in Chapter 5 as part of the social aetiology of illness. But, of course, the reaction to illness – that may make things worse – is also part of the patient's coping strategy. Particular examples of these strategies can be found in the patient's response to stigma and to being institutionalized.

MANAGING STIGMA

Goffman suggested that a person with a stigmatizing condition could pursue several coping strategies that were largely based on the salience of the stigma he or she carried (Goffman 1963). On the one hand, the stigma could be very obvious to others and therefore be a *discrediting* attribute; or, on the other hand, it might be relatively hidden and therefore be *discreditable*. A patient with a discrediting attribute has only a limited range of options because the stigma is present for all to see; a patient with a discreditable attribute, however, has the option of trying to keep the stigma concealed.

- *Passing*. A person with a discreditable stigma can try to pass as 'normal'. Depending on the medical problem, this will often require various forms of subterfuge, with the constant risk of exposure. This threat of disclosure and possible shame can be a constant source of psychological tension. For example, patients with colostomies may worry about their bag leaking whenever they go out or visit friends: their concern rests on the embarrassment and disclosure that such an event would produce.
- *Covering*. A person with a discrediting attribute has no opportunity to pass,

but can still try to minimize the significance of his or her stigma. This may be by avoiding situations in which the stigma would be revealed, or by reducing the visibility of the problem that is stigmatized. For example, cosmetics can cover, literally, many facial stigmata.

- *Withdrawal.* The avoidance of difficult social situations can be taken further by deliberately withdrawing from social life. In this way, the stigmatized person avoids all contacts that might produce embarrassment or shame.

In Goffman's analysis, all stigmatized people wish to hide away their shameful marks; moreover, he presents a stigmatized attribute as something a person has or does not have. More recent studies, however (described below), suggest that the picture is not so clear: some people, for example, deliberately 'come out' with their disabilities, whereas others are never sure from one day to the next whether they have a stigmatizing attribute or not. Even so, the coping strategies that Goffman outlines are a useful way of understanding some of the ways in which people manage labels.

INSTITUTIONALIZATION

A particular variant of secondary deviance is the process known as 'institutionalization' (Jones and Fowles 1984; see also Chapter 5). It is now well established that if people are placed for many years in a large impersonal institution such as a prison or a mental hospital, their attitudes and behaviour change. In an institution, with its own set of rules and routines, inmate behaviour, however resistant at first, will gradually change towards conformity, if only to make the daily routine more manageable (Goffman 1961).

The process of conforming is often considerably aided by institutional practices that have the effect of 'depersonalizing' the inmate on first admission. Personal effects are rarely allowed and private space or activities are kept to a minimum. The effect is to reinforce the exclusion of the inmate's 'old' self and the emergence of a new institutionalized identity. Inmates must adjust to new routines of sleeping, eating, relaxing, defaecating etc., which have often been introduced more for the benefit of the staff and institution than for the needs of the patients. (Because of the difficulties for staff in identifying short-term goals in chronic care, many seem to resort to 'goal displacement', in which the rather general and non-specific end-point of 'care' gets displaced in favour of specific short-term targets such as finishing meals by a certain time or ensuring that the laundry is efficiently managed.)

The problem with this new identity and patient readjustment is that, although they might facilitate institutional existence, they are inappropriate for life outside. In particular, the dependency that institutions create in their inmates means that they may have great difficulty in adapting to independence outside the walls of the institution. The problem of dependence is, of course, exacerbated by the fact that most of those hospitalized for a long period are precisely those who, through mental or physical impairment, were unable to cope on their own.

These effects are well known and there is now a policy to try to prevent institutionalization by keeping people in the community for long-term treatment – though the effectiveness and rationale for this have been challenged (Scull 1977). Otherwise, some of the effects of institutions can be minimized by trying to reduce some of the more stark, depersonalizing features of an institutional atmosphere. Furthermore, even when treatment does require lengthy hospitalisation, specific attention can be directed towards maintaining or re-establishing the patient's autonomy through forms of mental and physical rehabilitation.

COPING WITH CHRONIC ILLNESS

The labelling perspective laid the foundations for a fundamentally social view of disability by arguing that the doctor's answer to the medical question 'What is it (the disease)?' could also become the patient's answer to their question 'Who am I?'. Thus a medical diagnosis, accurate and made in good faith, could become the new 'master' identity for the patient. Such new identities were deviant ones, so patients had to contend with the role of social outcast.

While helping to explain the effects of illness on the patient, the labelling perspective can become too mechanistic, implying that labels produced their effects with minimal involvement of the patients; indeed, it seems less the label itself that is of importance than the reaction to it (which might even be to an 'imagined' label). In addition, labelling can seem a limited explanation for patients' reactions to illness: certainly, people respond to stimuli/labels, but why do certain labels have this effect and not others, and why do some people produce a greater reaction than others? The sociological answer has been an increasing attention to patients' meanings and, with it, new methods of research.

Very broadly, there are two ways of approaching the study of human behaviour. The first, taking its cue from the natural sciences, is to seek explanation in terms of causes. For example, were labels held to 'cause' a response in the patient, a study might somehow measure labelling and the response and then examine the relationship between the two. This method assumes that human behaviour needs the same sorts of explanations that characterize biological diseases. The difficulty is that human behaviour is not the same type of phenomenon as, say, inflammation, not least because inflammation remains much the same whatever the measurement procedure, whereas a question to a patient on, say, their emotional well-being or the state of their marriage has already contaminated the result, because unlike inflammatory cells, people react to being investigated.

There are techniques available that attempt to minimize the methodological biases associated with researching a 'knowing subject', but then there is an even more fundamental conceptual difficulty – namely, the role of reasons and meaning in social life. Inflammation responds to stimuli that are somehow external to it, whereas people respond to meanings that are inherently internal. For example, while poor interpersonal relationships, anxiety or immobility may be seen as 'causes' of experiencing increased pain, the critic can argue that this is just a shorthand: what actually happens is that the patient interprets these events and it is the meanings given to them that are inseparable from the actual experience. All symptoms are percepts and intimately related to the human being as an interpreting animal.

This form of argument has led to the development of methods to investigate meanings. These methods tend to be ethnographic, treating each person as a stranger. The approach produces intensive descriptive studies of small groups of people, in each case trying to establish how the person makes sense of the world. Society is not 'out there', but inside people's heads; the social reaction can only therefore be studied by exploring this internalized social world. What do people make of the reaction of others? How do they manage? What does it mean to them? How do they go about answering the question: 'Who am I?'?

PATIENT MEANINGS

According to the labelling approach, in the act of diagnosis, medicine provides a master label to the patient, especially for disabled people. This simple view has been challenged by the claim that patient self-definition is an altogether more complex procedure than this (Safilios-Rothschild 1970). In interviews with a group of disabled people, it was found that disability seemed to have meanings and consequences for them that were different from those of a traditional 'illness' or 'disease'. Yet these views of disabled people were, by and large, ignored by the health professionals, who had *their* idea of what the disabled role should be and used their influence to persuade the disabled to accept it. Indeed, the disabled were like any minority group who had their 'real' wishes and potential defined by others. Health professionals make judgements on behalf of the disabled without asking the individuals about their problems, preferred solutions and alternatives, or by openly disregarding all information received from the disabled individuals themselves about desirable goals (Safilios-Rothschild 1976).

The complexities surrounding the development of disabled peoples' self-perception were further explored by Blaxter (1976) in a study of 194 physically impaired patients. She found that the whole question of who was disabled could not be answered as neatly as had been assumed, because the boundary between disabled and non-disabled seemed constantly blurred, both at the 'official' level and, more importantly, at the level of self-definition. Further, the health and welfare services did not produce a massive and overwhelming 'labelling' effect, because they themselves were confused about who was to count as 'disabled'. In part, this was because of important differences in the way different health and social care workers classified disability, but also because of uncertainty on the part of individual professionals as to whether a label of disability at a particular time would help or harm the patient. Added to this, the so-called disabled themselves showed marked temporal variation in their own assessments of whether they really were disabled and/or its severity.

Accordingly, Blaxter argued that the disabled were not a homogeneous group and the 'label' to be affixed to someone was the result of negotiation between patient and professional. Patients could reject a label just as much as they could accept one; indeed, the identity of 'disabled' might change considerably over time. The important feature of this process, Blaxter suggested, was the patient's own 'constructions', which might be quite at variance with medical views; indeed, she found that patients' attempts to make sense of their illness often produced accounts markedly different from those in their medical records, and this could create problems in terms of adjustment and rehabilitation.

Goffman's analysis had suggested that disability was an unambiguous status, but for many diseases this assumption seems unwarranted in view of the ambivalent and changeable response of patients to the question of who they are. The very fact that the course of the disease and self-definition were uncertain on even a day-to-day basis meant that the strategies themselves had to be similarly varied, covering up one moment to avoid stigma or the threat of dependency, and eliciting help the next. The uncertainty about the course of the disease allowed the patient at one time to hope for relief or remission, while at another dreading a deterioration or relapse. In effect, as Weiner (1975) observed in a study of patients with rheumatoid arthritis, such patients were engaged in a continuous and precarious balancing of options. Every day was a mental trial. People did not 'adjust' or 'come to terms' with their disability as health care professionals might imagine; rather, they tried constantly to devise a viable strategy for getting through each and every day, continually varying their self-definitions to cope with the immediate problems of living.

COGNITIONS AND HEALTH

Health and social care agencies often define what disabled people 'need' in terms of services, but their ideas might be far removed from those of the patient. In her study of physically impaired patients, Blaxter identified several types of problem that related to activities of everyday living: problems to do with finding, maintaining and adjusting to work; money problems; and social problems associated with establishing and maintaining relationships (Blaxter 1976). Blaxter's analysis of the interviews enabled her to identify three-quarters of the sample as having at least one problem in one of her predefined areas in the survey year; of these, less than half were solved during the year. In consequence, she could conclude that there were real patient-defined needs going unmet in her population.

Blaxter's list of unmet needs was added to by a not dissimilar study by Locker (1983). Locker interviewed a sample of patients with rheumatoid arthritis. Like Blaxter, he was concerned with patients' self-definitions of their problems, but the 'problem areas' he identified were different in various ways. Following Blaxter, he found that occupational and relationship problems were important, as were practical difficulties of everyday living. Also, he identified the medical problems arising specifically from the disease, such as managing the drug regimen. In addition, he discovered the importance of the patients' struggle to attempt to make sense of the onset, course and future of the disorder and also their problems in understanding the workings of the medical and welfare agencies that offered treatment and social support.

The idea that patients' cognitions were important was relatively new. The traditional medical model would presumably claim that patients' knowledge of their illness came from directly experiencing it, and this knowledge, conceptualized as reports of symptoms, was a useful component of the medical history. Thereafter, the patient did not need knowledge other than to report symptom changes, as diagnosis and treatment could occur independently of the patient's own perceptions of the nature of the illness.

However, such a model of doctor–patient communication does not seem so applicable to chronic and disabling illnesses in which 'recovery' is not the norm. There is also recognition that part of proper medical management requires the provision of an explanation. It was not simply a case of telling everything, in that doctors resort to what Blaxter referred to as 'information management'. Because of the frequent clinical uncertainty of both diagnosis and prognosis, doctors feel constrained to control the amount of explanation given to the patient at any point in time. Equally, certain information is withheld from the patient as part of the overall case management. Information transfer has thereby become one of the therapeutic tools in an often-limited range.

Locker's study identified a further facet of the exchange of knowledge between doctor and patient that was not restricted to patients reporting symptoms and doctors providing explanations. Patients possess 'lay theories' or 'explanatory models' of their illnesses that are, in their own terms, as coherent and sophisticated as medical theories (see Chapter 2). True, medicine might view some aspect of the patient's theory as mistaken, but are the criteria medicine uses to identify truth and error the same as or wholly relevant to patients? Moreover, at a practical level, changing one element in a patient's cohesive theory by 'educating the patient' looks remarkably difficult to achieve.

Patient theories or cognitions are also important in their implications for an effective and harmonious doctor–patient interaction. As Locker argued, cognitions become one of the resources that the chronically sick and disabled possess. In effect, physical impairment and social handicap are not linked simply through the reactions of others (see Chapter 5), but also through the patient's own cognitions. Thus it is possible to distinguish 'enacted' or experienced stigma from 'felt' stigma in that it is not the social reaction that produces social disability but the disabled person's own self-perceptions of those reactions (Scambler 1984).

In the light of these cognitive models, the problem of coping with disability and self-identity can be seen differently. In Bury's (1982) study of another group of patients with rheumatoid arthritis, he again noted the day-to-day struggle to cope with the disease, characterizing its principal effects on a wider canvas as 'biographical disruption'. Bury argued that the 'taken-for-granted' assumptions and commonsense boundaries that everyone establishes to make life manageable are breached by some patients. Not only has everyday life to be renegotiated, but also the disruption to 'explanatory systems' used by everyone else requires a fundamental re-thinking of the disabled person's own biography and self-concepts, which in its turn throws into relief the cognitive and material resources available to the individual.

Contrary to the usual criticism of the biomedical model as ignoring the psychosocial identity of the patient, Bury suggested that the otherwise limited medical explanation was an important cognitive resource for the patient. The very fact that doctors, by and large, failed to move away from the 'it' of disease meant that disease was held separate from self. This enabled disease to be maintained at a distance, so that patients could claim that they were the victims of external forces; patients could answer the question 'Why me?' without the additional burden of responsibility or guilt. True, medical explanation and understanding were both ambiguous and limited, but they still provided at least one relatively fixed point on a terrain of uncertainty.

Other researchers have emphasized the impact on self-identity of an illness, especially a chronic one. Charmaz (1983), for example, explained the impact of suffering in terms of 'loss of self', in that many patients with chronic illness suffer a sort of bereavement reaction to the death of their old identities. Also, Williams (1984) provided a similar analysis when he pointed to the idea of 'narrative reconstruction' as the key process ill patients need to go through as they try to make sense of their own life stories and the place of illness within them.

In a study of patients being treated for cancer, none denied the diagnosis, yet, at the same time, many reported themselves as healthy (Kagawa-Singer 1993). These patients saw themselves as capable, competent, productive and valued by friends and relatives: their sense of self-integrity was therefore intact and in these terms they were healthy, despite their poor medical prognosis. From this point of view, the conventional medical judgements of health and illness need to be placed in the context of patients' own evaluations and coping strategies.

EXPERTS' MEANING SYSTEMS

Blaming doctors for giving diagnostic labels has largely disappeared, not least because labels can provide an important coping resource for the patient as well as a damaging marker. Equally, recognition through the World Health Organization's original classification of impairments, disabilities and handicaps that social reactions can have very real effects on patient identity and self-definition has been tempered by the criticisms of the disabled themselves (see Chapter 5). Experts, following the traditional medical model of disease (see Chapter 9), often use an individualistic approach to understanding the problems of coping with illness when they should also be looking to the social environment as a potent source of both potential support and harms. The task is to steer a difficult course between providing help and support, and creating dependency and devalued status.

Medical explanation can form a valued component of how the disabled make sense of their lives, but it would be a mistake to imagine that this is an injunction to 'tell all' to the patient. If recent work in sociology has shown anything, it is the complexity and sophistication of patients' explanatory models and meaning systems. These seem to lie at the heart of how patients cope with their illness on a day-to-day basis. As has been argued in a different setting (Tuckett et al. 1985), there is a case for doctors to recognize that their consultations are settings in which explanatory models are exchanged. In this light, use of listening and counselling techniques to elicit their patients' cognitions may further help their patients to live on a day-to-day basis with their illnesses.

CARERS AND COPING

Illness, as the previous section describes, has fundamental effects on patients. Not only is their biological functioning impaired in some way, but their psychological and social worlds are disrupted and need constant managing. It is clear that illness is as much a psychosocial phenomenon as a biological one.

In some ways, illness can be seen as ripples on a pond: the biological lesion causes upset to the patient's psychosocial adjustment, but then it moves further out to touch people close to the patient, particularly his or her immediate carers. Many patients with chronic and debilitating illnesses are very dependent on others for physical and psychological support, and the significant role of these carers in helping the ill cope is now well recognized (see also Chapter 10). What is less well understood is the impact of the patient's illness – both its biological nature and its psychosocial reaction – on the health of carers. The little evidence that exists would suggest major problems with the health of carers as they struggle themselves to cope with an illness that is located in another's body (Lewis and Meredith 1988; Glendinning 1992). Interestingly, it seems that it is less practical tasks and more interference with social life that are more important for carers (Jones and Vetter 1985). Nearly one-quarter of carers of patients with a stroke described social isolation or restriction as their most distressing problem; and carers were also particularly upset by changes in the patient's mood, no doubt reflecting their emotional involvement with the patient (Anderson 1988).

Chapter 9

MODELS OF ILLNESS

The preceding chapters in this book illustrate the extent to which the strict bio-medical model is a limited interpretation of the nature of illness. This chapter consolidates this perspective by an examination of the explanatory power of the biomedical model through a closer examination of one common patient complaint, abdominal pain.

EXPLORING ABDOMINAL PAIN

When confronted by a pattern of signs and symptoms in a patient, medicine constructs a differential diagnosis, a list of the pathological lesions that would produce such a clinical picture. For example, for a patient presenting with abdominal pain, there is an assumption that something in the abdomen is causing the discharge of afferent nerve fibres. The possible origins of the pain include pathological processes such as inflammation and ischaemia. The history of the pain together with abdominal examination usually lead to a diagnosis: if the pain is acute, it may indicate appendicitis caused by inflammation of the appendix; chronic pain, on the other hand, is usually more associated with ulcers or diverticulitis, though there are many other abdominal diseases in the differential diagnosis such as cholecystitis, Crohn's disease, ulcerative colitis etc.

ABDOMINAL PAIN IN CHILDREN

Various studies have looked at the incidence and diagnoses of abdominal pain in children. Such pain is fairly common, yet it is unusual to find an organic pathological basis for it.

One typical study based in general practice collected all the cases of abdominal pain in children presenting over a 7- year period (Turner 1978). The sample eventually amounted to 162 children, who were investigated as appropriate. Five were found to have a possible organic basis for their pain, which meant that the other 157 had pain of unexplained origin. Medicine often groups diagnoses in this latter group together and gives them the label of functional or idiopathic pains, precisely because their origin is unknown.

However, the study in question tried to explore the wider ramifications of the pain by comparing the close relatives of the children with abdominal pain with a control group. It was found that the close relatives of children with abdominal pain:

- consulted more frequently,
- had more abdominal pain and abdominal operations,
- had higher rates of psychiatric illness and referral,
- had more known marital problems.

These findings suggest various hypotheses about the basis of the pain.

- Many children in the community have abdominal pain, but the amount that is taken to the doctor will very much depend on parental response to the symptoms. If parents are high consulters, then, by and large, they have a higher likelihood of bringing their children's abdominal pain to the doctor. This may well help to explain the higher consultation rates of the parents and relatives of children with abdominal pain.
- The fact that the parents and relatives themselves have more abdominal pain might suggest two explanations for the child's pain: the child observes the abdominal symptoms in the parents and for various reasons mimics them; or, alternatively, the parents, having experienced abdominal pains, may now be more alert to similar problems in their children.
- The higher rates of psychiatric illness and referral observed in the close relatives of children presenting with abdominal pain compared with the control group might suggest either that the child is responding with 'belly aches' to a parent's psychiatric problems, or that the presentation of the child is itself a symptom of the psychiatric illness in the parent. In other words, the real patient is not the child, but the parent or relative.
- Similar explanations might apply to the observation that more known marital problems were presented in the close relatives of children with abdominal pain. Either the child is responding to the marital difficulties with pain, or the parents are using the child's illness as a way of showing their own problems: perhaps the child can provide a ticket of entry to the doctor.

In each of these possible explanations, the basis of the illness moves from its apparent location in the child's abdomen to the relationships within the family. This supports other well-established evidence that family dynamics are bound up with illness (Meyer and Haggerty 1962).

LIFE EVENTS AND APPENDICITIS

One hundred and nineteen patients between the ages of 17 and 30 presenting with appendicitis and undergoing appendicectomy together with a similar number of controls were interviewed about life events in the previous year. The total number of events was noted, as was the number classified as 'threatening' and 'severe' (Creed 1981).

After these interviews had been completed, the pathological reports on the state of the appendix were read. Sixty-three of the appendices (about half) were inflamed and the others were normal. However, when this pathological appearance of the appendix was linked to the life events experienced by the patient, an interesting picture emerged. Patients experiencing a severe life event (such as a bereavement of a close relative) in the preceding year were much more likely to have a non-inflamed appendix compared with the rest. In fact, the proportion of patients with normal appendices having severe events was remarkably similar to the percentage of patients who were found, in a different study (Brown and Harris 1978), to be depressed after experiencing severe life events. In addition, compared with a control group, even those patients with a pathologically inflamed appendix showed a much higher rate of threatening life events.

Surgeons are not able to predict accurately the pathological appearance of the appendix; they simply operate when they diagnose a likely inflamed appendix. It is well established, however, that about half of all appendices taken out are 'normal', despite the patient having shown all the clinical signs and symptoms of appendicitis. So why do patients get appendicitis, real or apparent? In this study the microscopic appearance of the appendix was somehow linked to the life experiences of the patients in the preceding year. Having a severe life event seemed to be related to having an apparent appendicitis in the same way that it was linked to the onset of depression. In fact, when the patients' psychiatric state was assessed, depression rates amongst the non-inflamed appendix patients were twice the rate amongst controls and the inflamed. In other words, it seemed that a severe life event may bring about depression, appendicitis or both. The pain of appendicitis would appear to have emerged as much from negative life experiences as from the nerve fibres of the abdomen.

LIFE EVENTS AND GASTROINTESTINAL DISORDER

A study of life events and gastrointestinal disorder investigated the relationship between patients with abdominal pain referred by general practitioners (GPs) to gastrointestinal clinics and preceding life events (Craig and Brown 1984). The proportion of patients reporting life events was then examined amongst those patients who were shown to have an 'organic' basis for their pain, those without ('functional' pain), and those in the control group. Numbers experiencing a severe life event in the preceding 38 weeks were 23 per cent, 57 per cent and 15 per cent, respectively. In other words, severe events seemed, as in the study described above, to be linked with abdominal pain of unexplained origin. Also, as in the previous study, there seemed to be a link between severe events and actual pathological lesions inside the abdomen. The pain was located in the abdomen, but the illness, it seemed, was to be found elsewhere.

The traditional model of medicine explains symptoms by trying to identify their origins in a pathological lesion inside the body. The doctor does this by identifying signs, carrying out relevant investigations and making a diagnosis. However, each of the above three studies showed that in many cases the exact nature of the illness could not be diagnosed by simply examining the inside of the body. The disease did not exist under the skin but in the patient's environment, psychological state, coping strategies, social relationships etc. Symptoms do not necessarily indicate a biological, pathological lesion and health care needs to attend to a wider psychosocial context if it wants to reach an understanding of the nature of the patient's problem.

SYMPTOMS AND PATHOLOGY

Further support for a different view of symptoms from that advanced by a strictly biomedical model comes from a variety of sources, including the results of screening programmes.

In an attempt to uncover some of the 'clinical iceberg' in the community, medicine has devised screening programmes through which to identify previously unrecognized diseases. Sometimes these screening exercises have involved checking for symptoms as indicators of underlying pathology – the implication being, as in traditional biomedicine, that the symptom is present because a disease is also present. To test this assumption, epidemiologists usually compare the symptom uncovered by the screening test with more certain evidence for the existence of the disease (by a reference test).

For example, in trying to determine the extent of urinary tract infections in women in the community, it is possible to use the presence of dysuria (pain or a burning sensation on micturition), one of the classic symptoms of urinary tract infection, as the screening test. Would this be adequate? The answer can be found by comparing the results of this screening test with the results of a reference test – namely, the presence of bacteria in a midstream urine sample (MSU).

When the results of such a symptom check are linked with the results of the pathological test, an interesting picture emerges (Komaroff 1984). First, there are, of course, some patients who experience dysuria and who have a positive MSU and who therefore can be said to have urinary tract infection, as well as patients with neither symptoms nor bacteria. On the other hand, somewhat surprisingly, there are some patients who experience the symptoms of urinary tract infection, but whose urine is sterile. The exact origins of the pain on micturition are unclear, but it would not appear to be due to urinary tract infection. Then there is a large group of patients who are asymptomatic, experiencing no dysuria, yet who have positive MSU results.

How are these results to be interpreted? There may be some laboratory failings, but the magnitude of the picture suggests something else is happening. The classical medical model would indicate that there should be a close correlation between symptoms and the pathological findings of disease. However, such studies of the prevalence of urinary tract infections show there are considerably more women with only one of the dyad than with both. It is difficult to say whether, in fact, such women really have a disease, as the exact nature of the disease is uncertain.

The implications of this for the medical model is that the supposed correlation between symptoms and pathology is not as clear-cut as it might seem. For example, patients may experience an anginal type of chest pain, yet the coronary arteriogram shows no narrowing of the coronary arteries. Have these patients got angina? Technically, no, because they have no narrowing of their coronaries. Yet they still experience the symptoms of the disease. So what exactly does the symptom mean if it occurs independently of underlying pathological change? It does at least suggest that the traditional biomedical model, which would relate all symptoms to pathological change, is inadequate for explaining the phenomenon.

The weakness of the biomedical model in these situations is not merely a theoretical one, in that it does also have real implications. For example, a third of patients with angina waiting for coronary artery surgery have psychiatric morbidity before the operation; afterwards, these patients remain disturbed, and their angina and exercise tolerance improve less than in those patients without psychiatric illness beforehand (Channer et al. 1988). To put it bluntly, a surgical operation is unlikely to be effective if the problem is not located in a patient's anatomy.

BIOGRAPHICAL OR PATIENT-CENTRED MEDICINE

Many GPs have observed that their patients have symptoms of disease, as described above, yet on investigation have no apparent pathology. This not uncommon situation has led many GPs to think about the character of their work and the nature of illness. One famous attempt was that provided by Michael Balint (1964). He was trained in both medicine and psychoanalysis and attempted to combine the two. He recognized that many of the problems presented by patients in general practice did not have an organic basis, despite mimicking traditional physical disease. He concluded from this that illness was a psychosocial phenomenon as much as a biological one and that this perspective had several important implications for the GP's role.

- First, the GP's task was not to diagnose and treat biological disease, but 'to organise unorganised illness'. Patients presented with disorganized illness: they had abdominal pain, they had domestic problems, they had experienced a severe life event. The doctor's task in these circumstances was to organize these disparate elements into a coherent picture that would explain the patient's experiences. This may have involved treating the abdominal pain, but also recognizing that it was only one component of the overall diagnosis and treatment of the problem.
- Balint also felt that traditional therapeutics was limited. Drugs to change the biological functioning of the body seemed of limited applicability, given that very often the problem was not biological in nature. Besides, it is well known that half of patients do not comply with the drugs given by the doctor; indeed, perhaps 20 per cent of patients do not even cash the prescription the doctor gives them. In the light of this, Balint argued that the most powerful therapeutic tool the doctor possessed was himself or herself. Patients came to the doctor to get a 'dose of doctor'. In simple terms, this can be seen as a sort of

placebo, but the doctor had to recognize that it was not the technical medication but the human relationship that had the most effect on patients' welfare. Balint also pointed out that this drug – doctor – was poorly understood: little was known, for example, of the correct dosages, of its addictive properties or of its side effects.

- The third facet of general practice that Balint identified was the mutual investment that doctor and patient placed in their relationship. A consultation in general practice was not a single episode in which a doctor treated a disease. The individual consultation was one in a series of consultations that occurred over a lifetime. In other words, each consultation followed on from the next in a sort of 'extended' consultation. As the doctor got to know more and more about the patients – their biography, their relationships, their social and physical environment – he or she was better able to use the time of each new consultation more effectively and to develop a greater insight into the patients' needs. At the same time, the consultation and this developing relationship also afforded an opportunity to develop insight into the doctor's own needs. In other words, the relationship between doctor and patient was a mutual investment that, over time, should benefit both.

Balint's ideas were received sympathetically by many GPs, who were aware of some of the complex reasons why patients consulted with them. They also knew that the scope for using the classical biomedical model was more limited in general practice than in hospitals because of the very different morbidity spectrum. For example, every year the average GP will see about 600 patients with upper respiratory tract infection (of which most are viral), 375 patients with non-specific symptoms and only two patients with lung cancer (the commonest cancer). Even more rare are conditions such as phenylketonuria, which would require over 200 years in practice to see just one case (Fry 1983)!

Realization that the patient's world was as much a part of understanding and managing the patient's illness has led to the emergence of what is called 'patient-centred medicine'. This approach acknowledges it is the patient not the illness that should be the primary focus of medicine. The task is not to elicit symptoms and signs and make a clever diagnosis, but to listen to the patient to identify what the 'real' problem actually is. Then it requires some shared decision-making between doctor and patient to determine the best course of action. To be sure, the doctor has expertise to contribute to this discussion, but so has the patient, and if both parties are agreed, it is more likely that appropriate management of the problem will be given and that patient adherence will be high. Further, this way of practising medicine, it is argued, results in improved satisfaction for both patient and doctor (Mead and Bower 2000).

Patient-centred medicine remains an attractive (if sometimes poorly defined) way of offering health care. Arguably, it redresses some of the extreme imbalances of a system of medicine that treated the patient as a wholly biological system, but, equally, it may be possible to have too much patient-centredness. One reason a patient visits a doctor is to access medical skill and expertise and enable the doctor to shoulder some responsibility for taking care of the illness – an important facet of health care for patients who are ill and anxious. However, taken to extremes, 'shared decision-making' could all too easily involve the doctor persuading the patient to take responsibility for the risks of illness and its treatment, when in fact that can and should be an important part of the role of medicine.

SURVEILLANCE MEDICINE

In the eighteenth century the symptom was the illness. If a patient had abdominal or chest pain, that meant the diagnosis was abdominal pain or chest pain. Elements of this system of medicine still exist in psychiatry (the symptom of being depressed, for example, means the patient has depression) and in general practice (a sore throat or a headache usually signifies nothing more than that the patient has a sore throat or a headache). However, at the end of the eighteenth and beginning of the nineteenth century, a new system emerged that claimed that the symptom was no longer the illness but merely a pointer or indicator.

The new medicine of the nineteenth century – often referred to as biomedicine or hospital medicine or pathological medicine – introduced the revolutionary new idea that illness was a pathological lesion inside the body. This pathology produced symptoms – better to identify it by – but also signs, the marks of the pathology that the skilled clinician could elicit. Symptoms and signs allowed the (hidden) pathology to be diagnosed and appropriate treatment instigated. Alongside this new form of clinical practice emerged new techniques for exploring the patient's body, such as the clinical examination and post mortem, and a new place in which to apply them, the hospital.

For 200 years, this medical model of illness was dominant, as bodies were examined, new investigative techniques invented and hospitals proliferated. But then, in the closing decades of the twentieth century, a new way of thinking about illness emerged that might be called 'surveillance medicine' (Armstrong 1995).

Surveillance medicine focuses on the risk factor. In fact, all the elements of biomedicine – symptom, sign, investigation results, pathology – can be reconstrued as risk factors, as pointing to the chance of an illness in the future. Also, new additions such as lifestyle, health behaviours, social circumstances, genetic make-up etc. can be added to the list. Together, these allow a risk profile to be constructed for everyone, not just supposedly ill patients. In consequence, everyone is 'at risk' and therefore everyone hovers precariously between health and illness.

A visit to the doctor becomes a way of reassessing risk profiles, as one 'illness' causes the risks of others to be revised. This is best illustrated by screening, which often does not identify illness as such but rather changes in the individual's risk of getting ill. Much of illness prevention and health promotion is also about changing circumstances so as to reduce future risk. Also, most treatment involves a risk calculation: for example, the results of clinical trials are often presented in the form of the number of patients needed to treat so that one patient will benefit (the NNT statistic).

Arguably, this new form of clinical practice is spreading as more health promotion activity is encouraged, new techniques for risk calculation emerge and diseases such as diabetes are redefined as risk factors (in that they lead to other illnesses and complications). Its importance lies in the new way in which it requires medicine to think about illness and the fact that everyone is a target for the new surveillance techniques. This has led some critics to decry the 'medicalization' of everyday life, as more and more of our activities come within the purview of medicine and doctors seem to extend their control into areas of social functioning far beyond their traditional remit (see Chapter 15).

ALTERNATIVE MODELS OF ILLNESS

There is a growing demand for alternative therapies. Patients seem more willing to explore and use healing systems that employ different underlying models of illness, such as homeopathy, acupuncture, osteopathy etc. There are various reasons for this, but one of the factors seeming to influence this demand is the failure of biomedicine to address the full impact that illnesses have on patients (Sharma 1992). Traditional biomedicine simply addresses the pathological lesion, whereas illness affects the whole patient. If the doctor therefore limits his or her focus, the patient is likely to be dissatisfied and to seek help elsewhere.

MODELS OF THE DOCTOR–PATIENT RELATIONSHIP

THE LINK WITH BIOMEDICINE

Jewson (1976) argued that the relationship between doctor and patient has a very close correspondence with the model of illness that dominates at any time. In the eighteenth century, physicians were few in number and their patients mainly upper class and aristocratic. This status difference ensured the dominance of patients in the doctor–patient relationship such that doctors had to compete with each other to please the patient. The model of illness that emerged from this relationship was one based on the interpretation of individual symptoms (see above): doctors had no need to examine their patients; they only had to be attentive to their patients' demands and experiences (in the form of symptoms). The frequent use of this symptom-based model of illness, in its turn, ensured the maintenance of patient dominance in the relationship.

In the late eighteenth century, the hospital emerged as a place to treat the poor sick, initially in Paris, then later throughout Europe. Doctors now found themselves treating (usually for charity) socially inferior and therefore more passive patients. Jewson argued that out of these social relations a new medicine appeared that stressed not the symptom, but the accurate diagnosis of a pathological lesion deep inside the body. This new biomedical model of illness required only the presence of the patient's body and the clinical–anatomical knowledge of the doctor. In short, the new medicine emerged out of a relationship between a dominant doctor and a passive patient, and the practice of the new medicine, in its turn, reproduced precisely this relationship between doctor and patient.

CONSENSUAL MODELS

The biomedical model of illness and its related model of the dominant doctor in the doctor–patient relationship characterized the practice of medicine until the 1950s. The dominance of biomedicine was illustrated in any contemporary text on clinical method (Armstrong 1984), and the appropriate doctor–patient relationship can be seen in Parsons' formulation of the sick role (1951). The notion of the sick role was advanced to explain the formal network of mutual obligations and expectations that existed between doctor and patient (see Chapter 2). Within this schema, the doctor had a role that involved acting in the patient's medical interests; the patient's role was defined in terms of four specific characteristics: the patient gained temporary exemption from normal role responsibilities, the patient was not held responsible for his or her own illness, the patient must want to get well, and the patient should comply with legitimate medical advice.

Although there are some carrots in this relationship for the patient, the dominant picture to emerge was of a relatively passive and obedient patient. This would seem fully in accord with the requirements of the biomedical model.

By the late 1950s, however, particularly under the influence of psychoanalytic theories, a new dimension to illness – in the form of recognition of a psychological aspect – began to appear. It can be seen in the Balint view of general practice, outlined above, but also in a well-known typology of different forms of the doctor–patient relationship (Balint 1964).

Szasz and Hollender suggested that three types of doctor–patient relationship could be identified:

1 activity–passivity: in which the doctor is active and the patient is a passive recipient of medical treatment and advice;
2 co-operation–guidance: in which the doctor guides the patient, who co-operates;
3 mutual participation: in which both doctor and patient negotiate and share the crucial decisions.

Szasz and Hollender (1956) likened these types to different stages of childhood. Activity–passivity is equivalent to the relationship between a parent and a baby in which the baby is wholly dependent on the parent for everything. Co-operation–guidance is more akin to a parent and child relationship in which the child can respond yet must still rely on the overall guidance of the parent. Finally, mutual participation is said to mirror the relationship between adults; in this case both participants are autonomous and equal.

CONFLICT MODELS

Both Parsons' and Szasz and Hollender's models shared a consensual approach in that doctor and patient have a common agenda, because it was still ultimately the biomedical view that predominated. True, Szasz and Hollender advocated more mutual participation, but they assumed that this would be achieved in the context of a shared belief in the biomedical model. Yet all the while new psychosocial dimensions to illness were being explored and with them came a realization that the traditional consensus between doctor and patient was not inviolable. The interests of doctor and patient could diverge, and the doctor's biomedical interest in the patient's disease might not be entirely the same as the patient's interest in the wider impact of the disease on his or her life. This led various sociologists in the 1970s to propose a 'conflict' model of doctor–patient interaction in which competing perspectives could be acknowledged.

Freidson (1970) offered a broad critique of conventional doctor–patient relationships, pointing out that despite their apparent belief in consensus, they were all doctor-centred. In other words, the relationship was seen entirely in terms of what the doctor had to achieve – namely, biomedical diagnosis and treatment. Instead, Freidson argued there was a fundamental clash of perspectives between doctor and patient. For the doctor, the patient was simply another clinical case in a long stream of other cases; for the patient, on the other hand, the illness was a unique personal experience. These different perspectives led to potential conflict. Indeed, Freidson pointed out that the three types of doctor–patient relationship described by Szasz and Hollender were logically incomplete. If the doctor could have three roles – active, guiding and participating – then so too could the patient. This led him to propose the addition of two further 'types' to the original list. These were guidance–co-operation, in which the patient guided the doctor, who co-operated, and passivity–activity, in which the doctor was passive and the patient active. In other words, leadership in the consultation could fall to either doctor or patient.

NEGOTIATION MODELS

In recent years, the limitations of the traditional biomedical model have become more apparent. This process, together with the knowledge that patients have complex lay theories that they bring to the doctor (see Chapter 2), points to any conflict in the doctor–patient relationship being ultimately about models of illness. Put simply, the doctor has a biomedical view of illness, and the patient has a psychosocial one derived from his or her experience.

Many doctors, recognizing this inherent conflict, have turned to wider models of illness, and adopted new strategies in the consultation, particularly those that try to elicit the patient's views so that these perspectives can be addressed. Nevertheless, there is evidence that for many consultations doctors' narrow construction of the nature of the medical illness causes them to lose sight of the problems presented by the patient. For example, in a detailed study of 328 consultations in general practice, patients were interviewed after the consultation and asked what they could recall of what had happened and the advice given (Tuckett et al. 1985). It was found that patients were, by and large, able to remember the key points that the doctor made about the diagnosis, its significance and the appropriate action to be taken. However, although the key points could be remembered, fewer patients could actually make correct sense – as the doctor intended – of the consultation. When it came to looking at whether the patients were actually committed to the key points the doctor had made, the proportion of patients fell to about two-thirds. In short, a third of the patients could recall what the doctor had said but did not feel that the doctor's advice fitted the nature of the problem as they saw it.

These different models of the doctor–patient relationship and their evolution suggest that the nature of the relationship is intimately bound up with the way that illness is defined. As this chapter has shown, re-emphasizing points already made in previous chapters, illness can be construed in a variety of ways. Traditionally, biomedicine has been the dominant way of interpreting illness – that is, reducing it to a pathological lesion, and expecting compliance from patients. Increasingly, this view is seen to be too limited, and certainly would not appear to be entirely congruent with the patient's own interests, in which even non-compliance with medical advice may be a means of illness management on the part of the patient (Conrad 1985).

Chapter 10

TYPES OF HEALTH CARE

Symptoms and illnesses, as shown in Chapter 2, are very common in the community. In deciding on appropriate treatment, patients have a range of alternatives, from dealing with the symptoms themselves to obtaining professional help.

SELF-CARE

Given the sheer quantity of symptoms and illnesses experienced by people, it is apparent that most are treated by self-care. Most patients have knowledge of how to treat common conditions: a bruise, a cut, a headache, a bad cold etc. They supplement this expertise with various pharmacological preparations. It has been shown that the average household in Britain contains about ten different medicines (Dunnell and Cartwright 1972). Some of these have been prescribed by doctors in the past, and some have been obtained as over-the-counter medicines from the local pharmacist. These resources are widely used (Anderson 1979). There is evidence to suggest that people take, on average, at least two different medicines every week. Some studies have suggested that medicine taking is so high that in any 24-hour period about half the population will have swallowed some pharmacological preparation.

Some people who could look after themselves when ill, choose to use the health services instead. They therefore consume resources that could be devoted to people more in need. This logic has influenced health services – and the agencies that ultimately foot the bill – to encourage more self-care. This strategy seems particularly important when it comes to prevention, because it would seem that if people could be persuaded to follow healthy activities, this should diminish ill-health in the future.

Using a strategy to encourage self-care, particularly in the area of disease prevention, has clear advantages, both for people's health and for the future costs of health services. There are, however, two major problems that can arise if this policy is pursued too enthusiastically.

1 If people are persuaded to take responsibility for their health, there can be an unforeseen cost if they fail, because in a sense they are then responsible for their illness. This outcome has been called 'victim-blaming' because the victims of illness, instead of receiving sympathy and support, are offered blame

(Crawford 1977). Victim-blaming may be a particular problem for lower socio-economic groups, as they are least likely to be able to 'look after' their health, for reasons discussed in earlier chapters.

2 The other problem with giving people responsibility for their own health is that many individual measures are ineffective in the face of socio-structural causes of ill-health such as social class, poverty, unemployment etc. Moreover, an emphasis on the supposed value of individual measures deflects attention from wider social deprivation on to the individual (Kronenfeld 1979).

FAMILY CARE

While many people cope with illnesses by themselves, they also draw upon the resources of those living around them, often of necessity. Relatives, household members and friends can offer support and advice and a form of lay nursing if required. Most childhood illnesses, for example, are treated in this way.

THE FAMILY UNIT

Obtaining help and support from those living around usually means depending on the family unit. However, examining the extent and effectiveness of such family support depends on defining the family. On the one hand, it is all too 'familiar', and forms one of the basic building blocks of society; on the other hand, it turns out that this familiarity is more than likely founded on a rather mythical idealized family unit.

- *Historical origins.* It was a common belief that society before the Industrial Revolution was characterized by the *extended family*, which involved various relatives, beyond mother, father and children, living together in the same household. This pattern of family life was supposed to have given way in modern times to the *nuclear family*, which encompassed only parents and their immediate offspring.

  This view of a historical transition between two types of family structure misrepresented the past – as well as the present. Various historical demographic studies have shown that the nuclear family, far from being only a relatively recent development, was common in pre-industrial societies (Anderson 1980). Moreover, it would appear from studies of some traditional working-class communities that, although perhaps not restricted to the same dwelling place, the ties and interaction of the extended family still form a major part of community life to the present day.

- *Current structure.* The typical modern family is usually held to be mother, father and dependent children. However, from Table 10.1 it can be seen that if the current pattern of household formation in the UK is examined, the so-called typical family is not that common. Almost 60 per cent of households are made up of couples, but only 23 per cent contain a couple with dependent children. In short, only about a fifth of households contain the 'typical family'. Just

Table 10.1 Household formation in Britain

	Percentage of households	Percentage of persons
One person	29	12
Two or more unrelated adults	2	2
Couple		
With dependent child(ren)	23	39
With non-dependent child(ren)	6	8
No children	30	26
Lone parent		
With dependent child(ren)	7	9
With non-dependent child(ren)	3	3
Two or more families	1	2
	100%	100%

Average household size = 2.36 people.
After General Household Survey (OPCS 1998).

over one-quarter of all households are single person – many of them elderly – and 7 per cent are lone parents with dependent children.

It would seem, therefore, that it is difficult to generalize about the family simply because there is no such thing as a standard family (particularly as, even within the same apparent family structure, relationships can vary so much). For many analyses, the unit of the household is more useful than the family.

AVAILABILITY OF FAMILY CARE

The main role of the formal health care system is to look after people whose illnesses are too difficult or too serious to be managed solely within the home; but this demarcation is dependent on the adequacy of resources in both formal and household sectors. On the one hand, resources within the health care system are rarely adequate to cover completely all who need such care, so that many people with serious and debilitating conditions must 'cope' at home, perhaps with the help of a close relative. On the other hand, facilities, skills and support may be lacking in the home. Many ill people, especially the elderly who might benefit from care by their immediate families, are unable to obtain it, either because they do not live in a 'family unit' or because they have no-one available who might be in a position to offer support. In these circumstances, the patient must be either accepted into hospital (often as a so-called 'social admission') or found a place within another institution, such as an old people's home or nursing home, which can provide the resources and care that the patient's own home lacks.

One means of supporting care within the family is periodically to offer 'respite care'. This involves the ill or frail relative entering a home or hospital for a couple of weeks while the carer, so to speak, recharges his or her batteries. Such an arrangement allows committed carers to look after someone else while not allowing themselves to be completely overwhelmed.

COSTS OF FAMILY CARE

Having an ill person in the home can lead to extra expense: heating, lighting, cleaning, food, shopping, special facilities etc. These additional costs, which would otherwise be carried by the health service, are transferred to families that look after their ill members at home.

The largest additional cost, however, is more difficult to quantify and relates to the problems involved in finding someone within the family actually to do the caring. One of the traditional tasks for women, besides running the home, was to look after members of the family who fell ill (women themselves not being expected to become ill). However, with the changing role of women in contemporary society, more having full-time jobs, with perhaps more sharing of domestic tasks, an available carer is more difficult to find. Who should take time off work? Who should get up at night? What costs in terms of added tensions and friction within the home are incurred?

One of the problems is that we know so little about care in the home, its costs and its benefits. In many situations it might well be the best treatment; in others it might be inappropriate for either the well-being of the patient or domestic harmony. Comparison of 'home' versus 'hospital' treatment for various problems rarely attempts to evaluate these costs for the family. Despite our ignorance of the extent and limits of informal care, it would be wrong to take it for granted.

THE ROLE OF CARERS

The role of individual family or household members in looking after another has been recognized in the term 'carer'. Carers are particularly important because they carry a considerable load of caring that would otherwise fall on the health services. However, carers are often themselves elderly and often not in the best of health (see Chapter 8). There is also some evidence that the health of carers can be impaired by the heavy responsibility of providing what is often 24-hour care (Lewis and Meredith 1988; Glendinning 1992). This means that the health of carers is becoming an important concern for the formal providers of health care.

In that most ill-health is experienced by people on the lower rungs of the class structure, carers are more likely to be working-class women. Men and women aged under 45 from working-class families are more likely than their middle-class counterparts to provide care to an impaired or elderly person in the same household (whereas middle-class carers predominate when it comes to looking after someone in another household) (Arber and Ginn 1992).

COMMUNITY CARE

The importance of family and household care for many illnesses is clear, but, as pointed out above, such care can place great burdens on the family, and it assumes the existence of family members in some ideal setting who are willing and able to take on full caring functions. For many illnesses this supportive environment does not exist. However, if family care were to fail to support ill people in their own homes, overwhelming demands would be made on existing health care services. Thus the policy of many countries is to encourage home care, and support it with more resources from the formal health care system on a community basis: hence an emphasis on 'community care'.

The idea of community care emerged in the 1950s, particularly in response to the discharge of patients from large mental hospitals. In effect, community care then meant care *in* the community (in contrast to care in an institution). In recent years, however, the term has come to mean care *by* the community as the resources of the latter have been mobilized to help.

With adequate resources, general practitioners (GPs) can manage more health problems in the community without the patient being hospitalized. The community or district nurse can treat problems in the patient's own home that would otherwise have required hospital nursing care. Provision of home helps to look after domestic chores or meals-on-wheels to provide food can supplement family resources. Grants and benefits to those willing to stay at home and look after aged and incapacitated relatives can prevent such people from being permanently institutionalized.

These attempts to bolster the power of carers to look after more people in the community might be welcomed on the grounds that home care is generally preferable to the anonymity of hospital care. Nevertheless, several criticisms of community care deserve consideration.

- Community care is often under-funded. To a certain extent, formal and informal health care systems are complementary, such that if one system defaults the other tends to compensate. This apparent reciprocity between the systems, it has been argued, has been seized on by governments intent on containing expenditure on health care. One of the most expensive features of hospital care is the 'hotel' costs. Keeping patients in bed and providing them with services such as cleaning, heating, lighting, food etc. is very expensive, and if these costs can be removed by caring for people in their own homes in the community, considerable savings result. Thus it is possible to dispense with expensive hospital-based services by giving a vague and perhaps token commitment to community care. However, what in fact happens is that the increased resources going to community care are wholly inadequate and it is left to the family and individuals to pick up the pieces. Poor funding over many years also means that health professionals skilled in community care are in short supply.
- Community care requires co-ordination and collaboration between various health and welfare agencies. This liaison, for example between GP and social

worker, often does not exist, nor is it clear who should be responsible for organizing it.

- Professional interests tend to support the status quo, especially the pre-eminence of hospital funding. Encouraging community care usually means the re-allocation of resources away from the hospital sector, and for this reason is often resisted.
- Community care, by the community, depends on the willingness and ability of the community to cope. The burden usually falls on families, particularly their female members (see above). The role of women has been changing rapidly and it is becoming increasingly unreasonable to expect wives and daughters to devote themselves full time to the care of other members of the family unit.

The major difficulty with community care is therefore that it might produce a net saving and reduction in government spending, but there is a comparable (and hidden) additional cost falling on families with illness. Costs are therefore removed from the whole community (who ultimately fund government expenditure through their taxes) and placed on individual families with the illnesses, who may well be the least able to bear the increased demands.

Commitment to community care must therefore be seen in the context of who pays the costs – in all its forms – for this service. Community care, when adequately provided, is a very different phenomenon from when it over-relies on the informal care system – which might well be weighed down with its own problems.

SELF-HELP GROUPS

Some diseases and illnesses pose particular problems for care. Health professionals and lay carers provide treatment and help, but sometimes not of the right kind. This has led some patients with illnesses that produce very particular needs to group together to form their own communities or self-help groups. A self-help group enables the patient to obtain support and advice from others with similar conditions and, for many diseases and for many patients, this seems to be very important (Robinson and Henry 1977).

Self-help groups might be seen as filling in for health service deficiencies. For example, a doctor might treat multiple sclerosis as a particular debilitating disease, but for the patient who has to live with it 24 hours a day it is an overwhelming experience. Sharing this experience with others with the disease seems to be very helpful, both in terms of advice on physical problems and emotional support. Equally, sharing experiences of the disease can be seen as a sort of protest movement against a biomedical model that reduces illness to a pathological lesion. In multiple sclerosis, colostomy, epilepsy, diabetes and lots of other illnesses, the disease is more than the biological deficit, and self-help groups enable the wider context of illness to be made salient and appropriate help and support to be provided.

Self-help groups are often very successful. Their membership can number many thousands, and they often produce newsletters and hold meetings for their members. Over the years, some groups have been so successful that they have begun to organize themselves on more bureaucratic lines. They appoint a director, have a formal constitution, and raise funds for themselves and for research into their condition. The group comes to have specialized knowledge about the particular disease and, in sponsoring research, they can become influential in guiding treatment priorities.

As the process of acquiring expertise develops, the skills and knowledge of the self-help group start to rival those of doctors and this situation can lead to an ambivalent relationship with organized medicine. Sometimes the self-help group may recruit doctors to the organization for advice and help, but this immediately compromises the characteristic of the self-help group as a form of alternative medicine. Indeed, it is possible that the self-help group may simply be taken over by doctors and used as an extension of the health care system. These tensions are usually resolved in different ways. Some self-help groups become incorporated into medicine, with significant representation of medical professionals within the organization. Others choose to remain wholly independent of medicine, keeping their autonomy, yet losing any benefits that medicine might confer. Yet others exist in the tension between these two strategies: the medical profession is seen to be part of the solution, but it is also part of the problem.

PROFESSIONAL CARE

Professional care might be defined as that health care delivered by people in part-time or full-time employment in a health care capacity. Professions are an important type of occupation and their particular characteristics are described in the next chapter. However, in terms of the organization of health care, there are various subdivisions of professional care that can be made.

PRIMARY VERSUS SECONDARY

Most health services have evolved a system of specialization in which there are experts in particular types of illness. This has clear advantages for patients in that they can find someone with particular expertise of relevance to their problem. Medical specialization, however, creates two problems: first, there has to be a mechanism to ensure that patients and their illnesses are steered to the right specialist (as the patients themselves are unlikely to know the appropriate person); and second, it would be prohibitively expensive to treat all illnesses, especially minor ones, with specialist resources. This has led health care to be split between primary and secondary services.

Primary care
Primary care is provided for patients as a point of first contact with the health service (Starfield 1990). By its very nature, it must be generalist, being able to cope with whatever problems present. GPs are the traditional primary care doc-

tors, though in recent years they have increasingly become part of a primary care team, involving a wider range of health professionals and their respective skills.

If the problem warrants it, the patient can be transferred from the primary sector to the hospital-based secondary sector. In some countries, such as the USA, many doctors perform both roles, being primary care physicians and specialists in some branch of hospital medicine. This means the distinction between sectors is sometimes blurred. In Britain, on the other hand, for historical reasons (Honigsbaum 1979), there is a strong demarcation between general practice and hospital. This manifests itself in much less crossover between the two (GPs, for example, will rarely follow their patients into hospital) and as a rule, except in emergencies, patients' only access to the secondary sector is through a referral from a GP. In other countries, patients are at liberty to go directly to a specialist or a hospital if they choose. As the hospital sector is much more expensive than the primary care sector, this tends to mean lower health costs, other things being equal, in those countries such as Britain and the Netherlands that limit access to specialist services.

The idea that good primary health care is an effective and cheap means of managing most illnesses has not been lost on financially pressed health care systems. There is now general encouragement for doctors to go into primary health care, and there is a greater flow of resources into the sector to enable more and more illnesses to be treated in this way. Indeed, the World Health Organization has placed special emphasis on primary health care services, particularly in developing countries where funding is even more limited.

This emphasis on the importance of primary health care has further improved its status in the medical world. From being the sieve that separated out the 'interesting' cases for hospital referral, general practice has increasingly become a special type of medicine in its own right, often with its own distinctive models of illness (see Chapter 9).

Secondary care

Specialist services usually require access to beds and often expensive equipment; they therefore tend to be based in hospitals. On occasion, the technology is so complex and the knowledge base so esoteric that some of it is given a label of tertiary care. Secondary care is noteworthy for being expensive, and in recent years has been the focus of various strategies of cost containment (see Chapters 11 and 12).

Given the close relationship of secondary care with the institution of the hospital, an understanding of the former is intimately bound up with the history of the latter. The modern hospital first emerged in Paris at the end of the eighteenth century as the main place for doctors to use their new-found skills of clinical examination in the search for the pathological lesion. This new biomedicine prospered and so did hospitals. Hospital bed numbers in Britain grew continuously through the nineteenth and early twentieth centuries, reaching a peak about mid-century. Thereafter, there was a major decline, such that by the beginning of the twenty-first century there were less than a third of the number of beds that were available 40 years earlier.

In many ways the decline in bed numbers mirrored the massive decline in beds that occurred in the asylum system a few years earlier. In the middle of the twentieth century, about half of all hospital beds were for psychiatric patients; but then, quite suddenly, the big asylums were closed and most of their 'inmates' discharged into the community. Four explanations have been offered for this massive process of 'decarceration' (Scull 1977).

1 *Technological innovation.* The first argument is that the beds were closed because of the development of new drugs that suppressed psychotic symptoms (such as the phenothiazines) and enabled patients to live again in the community. However, it has been noted that the policy of decarceration began before the new drugs appeared. Technological innovation might therefore have furthered the policy of discharge, but it could not be responsible for it starting.

2 *The humanist challenge.* During the 1950s, a critique of the asylum system of care emerged that stressed:

- the inappropriate incarceration of many patients who did not need excluding from the community,
- the non-therapeutic and custodial nature of this supposed 'medical' care,
- the damaging effects ('institutionalization' – see Chapter 5) of being incarcerated for a long period of time (Goffman 1961).

This critique of the asylum system was supported by a broad anti-psychiatry movement that argued that whereas criminals at least had a hearing in court, mentally ill patients seemed to be incarcerated at the 'whim' of psychiatrists. Persecution of political dissidents in the old USSR under the guise of treating mental illness was used as an example, as was the behaviour of Western psychiatrists (Szasz 1962; Rosenhan 1973).

3 *Changing needs of late capitalism.* Scull argued that madness had first been subjected to asylum incarceration about the time of early capitalism as a means of controlling otherwise potentially disruptive and unproductive labourers. However, by the late twentieth century there were other methods available for handling unproductive labour, so the asylum system lost its main justification. Also, its costs were rising rapidly.

4 *Changing ideas about mental illness (and mental functioning).* The final explanation is that ideas about mental functioning changed to such an extent that madness became an outmoded label and, in consequence, the asylum became redundant (Armstrong 1979). In the nineteenth century, the only psychiatric disease was insanity, a problem of lack of reason afflicting the few who were then 'exiled' from normal society. In the twentieth century, a new group of mental illnesses emerged, the neuroses (anxiety and depression), which involved a problem in coping with emotions. Unlike madness, the neuroses potentially affected everyone and did not need managing in asylums.

Parallel arguments can be advanced for the subsequent decline of non-psychiatric hospital bed numbers.

1 *Technological innovation.* In the post-war years, there was an explosion of new drugs, new diagnostic techniques and new therapeutic techniques (Le Fanu 1999). These enabled more treatments to be offered as an out-patient rather than an in-patient.

2 *Changing views of hospitalization.* During the early twentieth century, the hospital bed was largely viewed as offering safety and therapy (through rest) for the patient. However, in the second half of the century these assumptions were challenged as the dangers of hospital stay and bed rest were discovered (Armstrong 1998). Thus, early 'mobilization' and early discharge became important facets of treatment. Even in the twenty-first century, the hospital continues to develop a reputation as a place where harm can come to patients just as much as benefit (Vincent et al. 2001).

3 *Cost containment.* In the latter half of the twentieth century, the costs of health care rose dramatically with the increasing demands of an ageing population, more expensive medical treatments and higher expectations from the population. One of the main costs was the 'hotel cost' of maintaining beds: one solution was to reduce in-patient care by moving to alternatives such as day care, 5-day wards, day surgery, and community alternatives.

The net effect of these various changes is that the hospital in the early twenty-first century is a very different animal from that in the mid-twentieth century. Ironically, while bed numbers have declined dramatically, the number of patients treated in hospitals has continued to rise. Fewer beds but more patients is explained by much shorter periods as an in-patient. Whereas 50 years ago a patient having a hernia repair might have stayed in hospital for 2 weeks, the operation is now most commonly conducted as day surgery.

ORTHODOX VERSUS UNORTHODOX

There has always been a struggle between orthodox and unorthodox healers. The orthodox, of course, is simply that group that has managed to seize the high ground – in Western medicine for the last 200 years that has meant biomedicine. Had phrenology won out in the nineteenth-century struggle for supremacy, medicine would look very different today.

Orthodox medicine protects its interests with two strategies.

1 *Marginalization* means that rival practitioners are excluded from regular medical work, often by labelling them as charlatans. Legislation in Britain in 1858 gave a legal basis to the medical profession's right to practise medicine and excluded many healers who used non-biomedical approaches.

2 *Incorporation* emerges when the unorthodox refuse to be marginalized. For example, in recent years the medical profession has shown a more liberal attitude towards unorthodox healers. Does this mean they are becoming more tolerant? Or is it a change in strategy? Perhaps, because these alternative medicines have increased their public support, it has been judged wiser to try to neutralize them through incorporating them into medicine than to allow

them the possibility of further independent growth (Sharma 1992). There is now the interesting spectacle of biomedical practitioners carrying out acupuncture, homeopathy etc., though often in a manner that would not win the approval of alternative practitioners themselves.

Whatever the impact of these inter-professional rivalries, there does seem to be an increasing trend towards using alternative medicines. Typical clientele of these services seem to be those with chronic pain, allergies, musculo-skeletal disorders and psychosomatic conditions who are disappointed with the care they receive from orthodox medicine (Moore et al. 1985). At the very least, alternative medicine practitioners seem to offer a listening ear and to take seriously the often intractable problems that some patients seem to endure.

PRIVATE VERSUS PUBLIC

There is a distinction between health services bought in a private negotiation between doctor and patient, and health services provided as a right, free at the point of use (Calnan et al. 1993). However, in most countries of the world this distinction is becoming increasingly blurred, as different political ideologies and economic imperatives jostle for influence over health care provision. These issues are dealt with in Chapter 12.

TEAMWORK VERSUS SOLO PRACTICE

Increasingly, health care is provided by groups rather than by individual health care professionals; in these teams the doctor is only one member. Efficient teamwork depends on good personal relations and a clear definition of what each member's responsibilities are. The professional aspirations of team members, however, can create various tensions. Occupational groups such as nurses and other paramedical groups are trying to achieve some autonomy from medicine, and this can lead to rivalries and ill-feeling. Further, because the new professional groups are trying to carve out a specific knowledge area, there can be clashes between neighbouring groups as to who possesses expertise in a certain situation. Who, for example, should take charge of caring for chronically ill people in the community? GPs, social workers, health visitors, district nurses etc. all have a claim to lead the health care team. However, each of these groups has a different knowledge base that at times overlaps with that of other members of the team, and at other times produces a different set of priorities and definitions of the situation.

Chapter 11

MEDICINE, THE PROFESSIONS AND CLINICAL AUTONOMY

One meaning of the term 'professional' is simply 'paid', in contrast to amateur. However, those occupations known as professions also hold more important social significance.

In the mid-twentieth century when sociologists first studied the nature of professional groups, they concluded that the professions offered a type of service that was quite distinct from that of other occupations (Goode 1960). Doctors were seen as an archetypal profession and their work was characterized by certain key features. One was a specialized knowledge base that patients needed. Another was a service ideal – that is, a commitment to the patient that went beyond simply doing a job for money. The three great professions, medicine, the law and the church, fitted this description well. Practitioners in each of these professions possessed specialized knowledge that was not easily accessible to lay people, and in addition they seemed to profess to be more interested in their clients' welfare than in their own.

In retrospect, it is now thought that sociological studies of the period too readily accepted the professions' own claims to expertise and altruism. A new, more sceptical, analysis of professions emerged in the 1970s that argued that these claims to a service ideal and esoteric knowledge were simply a form of rhetoric used in the pursuit of self-interest (Johnson 1972). Indeed, some analyses claimed that the history of the medical profession, in particular its exclusion of 'unqualified' lay practitioners in the nineteenth century, was less concerned with 'protecting the public' and more with self-interest and the creation of a very successful restrictive practice that has served doctors very well over the years.

The cornerstone of professional status is now believed to rest with the control such occupational groups have achieved over the content of their work (Freidson 1970). Doctors argue that this freedom from external constraint (or clinical autonomy) enables them to make judgements and direct resources in their patients' best interests. Critics, on the other hand, argue it gives doctors too much power to ride roughshod over the views (and real interests) of their patients and allows them to allocate large amounts of (often public) resources with minimal accountability.

The question of whether unfettered clinical autonomy is in the public interest became hotly debated in the closing years of the twentieth century. There were a number of problems.

- Numerous surveys of clinical practice uncovered wide variation in ways of managing the same illness. This would suggest that some patients were getting less than optimal treatment.
- Even when best practice had been established by research involving well-designed clinical trials, clinicians were very slow to change their old – and sometimes potentially harmful – habits.
- Consumerist society began to influence health care and patients increasingly demanded to be heard in the consultation and pursued redress when things had not gone to their satisfaction
- There had been a number of high-profile cases of medical negligence or even criminal behaviour. There was a strong argument that these had either occurred or been allowed to continue because doctors had been able to hide behind the idea of clinical autonomy, that they were acting in their patients' best interests and no-one should interfere. Further, medicine's own disciplinary bodies (operated by doctors because they are self-governing) had often failed to censure or punish clear breaches of clinical competence.
- Medical errors seemed relatively common (Vincent et al. 2001), but a culture of autonomy means that, for the most part, they remained hidden. Discussion and analysis of errors was used as an important learning opportunity by other organizations and, if it were not so defensive, medicine could have done the same.

The upshot of these various changes is that clinical autonomy and doctors' lack of accountability are under attack. Yet some freedom must remain if doctors are to exercise clinical judgement on behalf of their patients. How then to 'persuade' doctors to behave more 'responsibly'? How to 'control' doctors' wayward habits while allowing them discretion in the individual clinical encounter?

CONTROLLING INFORMATION

The basis of the medical profession's claim to work without supervision and accountability rests with its specialized knowledge. A hospital manager cannot tell a physician who to treat with a certain drug, nor would it appear easy without specialized surgical knowledge to reprimand a surgeon for operating unnecessarily. Knowledge and skill are therefore essential features of professional autonomy. Control over knowledge is thus one way of constraining a doctor's freedom.

TRAINING

If doctors are trained to act in a cost-effective way, it seems a reasonable hope that they will continue to do so throughout their professional lives. The problem is that medical education has traditionally been controlled by the profession itself, so the opportunity for external bodies to influence it has been limited. Nevertheless, governments usually control various aspects of funding, both of the training itself and in setting research priorities, which in their turn can influence the knowledge and emphases of medical education. Therefore, the potential is present for some direct intervention into the training of doctors, both in medical school and in later specialist and continuing education.

More important has been the ability of governments to control the accreditation and licensing of doctors. In the USA, states often control preliminary licensing, together with regular requirements for further and continuing education. In Britain, most education is controlled by the profession, but government influence is increasing. There is now a statutory requirement, for example, to complete 3 years of training before being eligible to be a general practitioner (GP) and there are financial credits for undertaking continuing education. A policy of re-accreditation, whereby doctors have to undergo regular assessment of their fitness to practise, is already common in many countries.

INFORMATION FEEDBACK

One of the arguments against clinical autonomy is that doctors are not accountable to anyone for their allocation of resources, but nor are they often aware of how much they are actually spending. The doctor decides a patient needs a blood test, an operation or a drug, and then provides it without knowing how much it costs. Clearly, in certain situations a service should be provided irrespective of the cost (though this is not true for all services that are 'needed', especially the very expensive ones). But equally, there are many situations in which, say, a particular test is not really necessary, or for which there is a cheaper alternative.

It follows that if doctors were made aware of the true costs of the services that they dispense, they would be able to make more cost-effective clinical decisions. This has led to an increasing flow of information to doctors informing them of the costs of decisions that they might make or have made. For example, British GPs are now supplied with monthly data on the numbers and costs of all their prescriptions, together with comparative data for costs in their locality and nationally. Thus GPs are in a position to know whether their prescribing is above or below the norms set by their colleagues, the assumption being that those with high costs will feel guilty enough to change their prescribing habits.

CLINICAL GUIDELINES AND PROTOCOLS

Evidence accumulates about best practice, often from clinical trials, but it is difficult for doctors to keep up with the amount of new research being published every year. One solution is to develop a clinical guideline or protocol describing the best management for a particular condition. Doctors sent the guideline would then be expected to conform to its advice unless there were special circumstances.

Despite the growing 'industry' involved with writing and distributing guidelines, the evidence suggests that they are not particularly influential on clinical practice. In part, this is because doctors get swamped by the number of guidelines they receive and sometimes they offer contradictory advice, but it is also likely that following guidelines is seen as too much like cookery-book medicine that does not allow individual practitioners to exercise the freedom and judgement for which they were trained and that they so value. The next step therefore is to make the 'guidance' compulsory.

LIMITING COSTS

Because of the uncertain nature of medical work, doctors cannot be told how much to spend on each patient. However, they can be given various overall constraints on expenditure.

LIMITED PRESCRIBING LISTS

Doctors need the freedom to prescribe the drugs that will benefit their patients. However, the costs of drugs to a health service are very high – more than 10 per cent of total expenditure – and it is generally believed that in many instances doctors prescribe expensive drugs when a cheaper one would work just as effectively. In part, this may be due to lack of knowledge of relative costs or of the similar pharmacological properties of a cheaper preparation; but in addition, a major part of continuing medical education is provided by the pharmaceutical industry, and it has a vested interest in persuading doctors to use expensive drugs while informing them of the benefits of its latest product.

Generic prescribing, in which only the generic drug names are used, would be considerably cheaper because, for those drugs out of patent protection, the proprietary product is usually a lot more expensive. However, again with the support of the pharmaceutical industry, doctors have resisted this change on the grounds that it is an unwarranted intrusion into their clinical autonomy to prescribe what they consider is best for their patients.

One response to the rising costs of prescribing has been to inform doctors of costs and relative pharmacological benefits. The other has been to limit the range of drugs that doctors are allowed to prescribe. Most hospitals now have limited prescribing lists in which only a restricted number of drugs is available. Alternatively, certain drugs – which are either ineffective or for which there are cheaper alternatives – can be placed on a 'black list' so that, if doctors wish to prescribe them, the patient must pay their full cost.

Some doctors have objected to these constraints as a threat to clinical freedom, but most have quietly accepted the restrictions. Indeed, doctors themselves have always been closely involved in drawing up these lists, and critics can hardly argue a very powerful case in favour of ineffective therapies. Nevertheless, many doctors see these limitations as the beginning of greater constraints on clinical freedom.

PREDETERMINED CARE

In the USA, health care costs have risen very rapidly (see Chapter 12). In response, a number of strategies have been developed that tend to predetermine the amount of resources that can be expended on any individual patient. Broadly, this involves assigning different clinical diagnoses with a financial allocation and expecting the clinician to manage within this constraint. Two specific techniques have emerged.

Diagnosis-related groups

A system of payment based on diagnosis-related groups has been introduced for many services as a means of containing costs through restricting the doctor's ability to spend. This is carried out by dividing all medical problems into about 500 'diagnosis-related groups' (DRGs), in which medical conditions that cost a similar amount to treat are grouped together. For each particular DRG, a fixed payment is made by whoever is footing the bill (government, insurance company, etc.). This encourages both the doctor and the hospital to restrain their expenditure to the expected amount they will receive. Some allowance is made for the fact that medical problems are unpredictable by permitting some increase in payment if there are either complications or other coexisting medical problems. However, to prevent providers making too many claims under these categories, their number is strictly limited.

Faced with these constraints, health care providers in the USA have pursued several strategies to try to minimize the restrictive effect of DRGs.

- There is the practice of shifting diagnostic categories – or 'DRG creep', as it is called. Hospitals and doctors have a bias towards making diagnoses for patients that carry a larger payment. Thus, if a myocardial infarction carries a higher payment than angina, it is in the provider's interest to make the former diagnosis rather than the latter.
- Because the payment that each DRG attracts is primarily based around length of bed stay in a hospital (this usually being the most expensive part of treatment), there is an incentive for early discharge of patients back to their homes and into the community. This, of course, simply shifts the costs of looking after illness from the hospital and/or doctor onto the community and the patient's own family. In certain circumstances, a 'failed' discharge can simply result in re-admission to hospital and a claim for another DRG payment.
- DRGs can lead to selection of patients. Certain DRGs are believed to offer under-payment and others over-payment. Thus, diagnostic conditions that tend to cost more than the agreed payment schedule will cause doctors and hospitals to run into loss. On the other hand, DRGs that carry a relatively large payment in terms of the usual costs of treatment will enable the doctor and hospital to make a profit. There is therefore an incentive to admit only those patients with particular diagnoses that are known to be covered by or to undershoot the appropriate DRG payment.

Managed care

Managed care works in a way similar to DRGs, but adds a list of the recommended care procedures to the financial constraint. This can prove even more constraining for clinicians, as clinical discretion is replaced by a relatively fixed protocol of care that needs to be followed if financial penalties are not to be incurred.

Clinical budgeting/management controls

The other, more general, method of cost containment is some sort of control over total clinical expenditure. This can be effected in a variety of ways.

Need-based budgets On a very general view, resources can be allocated to different geographical regions of a country on the basis of health need. Identifying health and health need is difficult (see Chapter 3), but after considering the various options, the British National Health Service (NHS) chose mortality as the best available measure (DHSS 1976). This meant that geographical areas were funded for health care on a formula based on capitation (a fixed amount for each individual in the area – often corrected for age and sex to reflect the higher health service demands made by the very young, the elderly and women) and local mortality rates. The correction factor for general practice funding in Britain is a measure of deprivation (derived from census data) that is meant better to indicate the higher demand made on primary health care in certain areas (e.g. inner cities). These overall budgets then provide a limit on the expenditure that can be incurred by the defined population.

Clinical budgets Another way of constraining expenditure is to give doctors themselves control over an annual (fixed) budget with responsibility to ensure that it is not overspent. Giving doctors direct responsibility for budgeting can be effective. First, they have far better information on costs, so they are potentially able to make more cost-effective decisions. Second, because they have control of allocations, they are better able to distribute the money over the required time period without running out at the end. Third, involving doctors increases their commitment to the notion of cost control: it is not a faceless manager dictating to doctors, but a means of maintaining – even enhancing – their clinical autonomy.

The major difficulty with clinical budgeting is that it requires doctors partly to become managers, as some of their time must be spent on financial management tasks. Besides the initial lack of skill and experience in this area, it means that doctors are drawn away from clinical work for an increased portion of their time. Doctors have had a highly specialized training in clinical work and it might seem inappropriate that much clinical output is 'lost' as they spend more time on management problems.

ECONOMIC INCENTIVES

Health care occurs in the wider context of a society's economic system. The 'market' economy that has been so successful in Western countries provides an essential backdrop for health care provision. If health care itself is provided by means of the market (see Chapter 12), the usual incentives and disincentives to carry out certain actions will apply. On the other hand, when health care is provided by direct government funding, there is a different set of priorities to provide a context for doctors' behaviour.

Economic incentives operate more directly on the different ways of paying the doctor. Compared with the overall costs of providing health care, the cost of paying doctors (who number about 5 per cent of all health personnel) is relatively small. Few costs would therefore be saved by restraining medical earnings – though no doubt doctors' pay forms a benchmark for other health service salaries. However, the method of paying the doctor does seem to have a major influence on health service expenditure above and beyond doctors' own pay, as well as on the type of service provided (Abel-Smith 1976). In effect, the method of paying the doctor acts as a financial incentive – or disincentive – towards certain types and styles of work.

There are basically three methods of reimbursing the doctor, and their relative advantages and disadvantages will be described, together with the influence they have on health costs and the definition of health need.

FEE-FOR-SERVICE

This is the usual method of payment in health care systems that tend to be dominated by 'private' funding and a market orientation (see Chapter 12). The doctor is paid a separate sum for each 'item' of service he or she provides. This method of payment is also found when insurance companies or governments intervene to cover patients for the costs of their care, the doctor charging them directly or indirectly for the services provided for insured patients.

The virtues of this system seem obvious. Doctors are paid, like many other skilled people, for the particular service they render. If they work hard, they receive a commensurate increase in income; if they choose to work only 2 days a week, they receive accordingly less. In short, fee-for-service acts as an incentive for doctors to work hard, as can be seen by the busyness of doctors (and dentists) paid this way.

In other industries, this piece-rate system may have much to commend it: the harder the labour force works, the greater the output and the larger the workers' incomes. Yet in providing health care to individual patients, the doctor's keenness to work might actually be counter-productive. Many medical problems may require the doctor to wait or be vigilant rather than be committed to speedy or heroic intervention.

Thus, although fee-for-service may be suitable for other occupations, it does raise problems in medicine. Given the doctor's claim to be able to identify health needs, it is the doctor who judges which service is necessary (not the consumer as in other situations) and thereby decides whether to collect a fee or not. In short, the doctor comes to have a vested interest in illness rather than in health. Slight menorrhagia, for example, may be more likely to become justification for an operation if gynaecologists will be paid extra money than if they will not.

Although there are professional and ethical pressures to prevent financial criteria from affecting medical decision-making, it has still proved necessary to organize widespread checks on medical practice when fee-for-service is the norm. In the USA, for example, peer review bodies will often assess the appropriateness of surgery in a hospital and bring pressure to bear on those who seem to be 'over-operating'. Peer group assessment, however, suffers from the potential bias that high intervention rates themselves become the norm in these situations. It is now well established that those health services that use fee-for-service carry our more medical procedures, examinations, investigations, operations etc. than those that do not.

Another example is afforded by the dental service within the British NHS, which mainly operates on a fee-for-service basis. A Dental Estimates Board approves fees for certain procedures and institutes random checks on the quality of work performed. Yet even this system can never exclude the possibility of unnecessary work being carried out. It has, for example, been suggested that a proportion of tooth cavities caused by caries would re-mineralize without treatment. However, in a fee-for-service system, the incentive is for the dentist to drill out and fill the cavity rather than to wait. Indeed, it is virtually impossible to check on a wholly unscrupulous dentist who 'fills' a non-existent cavity and claims payment for doing so.

Fee-for-service also leads to what economists call high 'transaction costs'. Whenever a 'service' is carried out – a consultation, X-ray, blood test – a fee must be claimed from someone. This means that systems dominated by fee-for-service have lots of claims being passed around at any time – which means a large bureaucracy to process them. Hospitals in the USA have large departments simply concerned with ensuring that fee claims are properly processed.

The other main problem with fee-for-service is that it can distort the definition of health need and health care by reducing health to procedures that can be itemized for payment. For certain parts of medical practice, this may be convenient, but for many patients' problems that need a wider definition of health (see Chapter 9), it tends to be inappropriate. Empathy, understanding and long-term emotional support, for example, are difficult to itemize and, indeed, even if they could be, their nature might well be changed: 'friendship-for-a-fee', for example, is very different from friendship.

CAPITATION

Capitation is a system in which the doctor is paid according to how many patients he or she looks after, irrespective of whether they use the service. Thus, two doctors with the same number of patients on their lists – and hence the same income – might work significantly different hours if one group of patients uses the service more than the other.

This system, in effect, works like the old Chinese method of paying the doctor, whereby the doctor was paid by patients when they were healthy and not paid when they were ill. The doctor therefore receives a higher income, relative to the work performed, the healthier the patient population. The key advantage of this system is that the doctor (as well as the patient) profits from good health, whereas under fee-for-service the doctor, ironically, benefits from ill-health. In principle, therefore, emphasis is placed on preventive measures, on support services and long-term care etc. in an effort to improve the general health of the population served. (In contrast, prevention under a fee-for-service system is in a somewhat ambivalent position because, although it might gain an immediate fee, it potentially reduces future earnings.)

One of the main problems with a system that works by encouraging current effort to improve patients' health is that such a strategy might not decrease future workload. There is not sufficient evidence to support the proposition that hard work by the doctor today will improve patients' health such that they consult less frequently in the future. Indeed, it has even been argued that the opposite effect holds: over-concern with patients and their problems merely makes them more dependent and even more likely to consult in future (see Chapter 13).

The other problem with capitation is that, instead of being concerned with improving patients' health for tomorrow, the doctor may come to be more concerned with how often they use the services offered today. In other words, low consultation rates, instead of being used as indicators of good health, become ends in themselves. The result is that if the doctor wishes to increase income relative to work input, there is an incentive to undertake the health care of too many patients and to give them only summary attention when they seek help.

A large component of the pay of British GPs is based on capitation. This means that they have lists of patients for whom they have taken responsibility to provide care. The GP is therefore in a position to provide continuity of care to this relatively fixed and well-defined population. This has not prevented the introduction of other techniques, based on both the stick and the carrot, to further encourage GPs to provide good quality services.

SALARY

The salary is, as it suggests, a fixed income irrespective of the work performed. It has the same advantages as capitation in that it acts as a disincentive to over-zealous and unnecessary investigation and treatment. Moreover, it has an advantage over the capitation system in that there is no incentive to take on more patients than can reasonably be managed (though 'excess' patients might then find themselves on waiting lists and in queues). However, it also has the same disadvantage in that there is no incentive to work hard. Even if there are fixed hours, the doctor has no financial encouragement to work quickly and efficiently within them.

OVERVIEW

When comparing systems of paying the doctor, it is as well to remember that, despite its undoubted appeal, money is not the only incentive behind good clinical practice. In the same way that the excesses of a fee-for-service system might be tempered by professional commitment to good medicine, so the disincentives in the capitation and salaried systems are often overcome by doctors' pride and satisfaction in providing good medical care. Rather than dictating practice, the method of payment tends to influence its emphasis, in particular how health need is defined and met.

In any health care system, it is not unusual to find a mixture of methods of payment that only illustrates the deficiencies of one or the other. Thus public health doctors are usually salaried, even in an otherwise fee-for-service system, and doctors paid by salary or capitation are often offered fees for specific services when these are deemed important enough to need encouraging, e.g. immunization or contraception.

Otherwise, the chief disadvantages with salary and capitation as methods of payment have to be contrasted with those of fee-for-service. To a certain extent, it might be argued that the tendency of capitation and salaried personnel to under-treat may be a more acceptable error than over-treatment, especially in view of the problems of effectiveness and efficiency of modern medicine (see Chapter 13). The other significant advantage of salary and capitation over fee-for-service is the relative cheapness of the former, both in terms of direct payments to doctors (the medical profession tends to do better from the latter) and in terms of the additional costs incurred by doctors' clinical decisions. This acts as an incentive for governments to adopt the cheaper system, and its greater ability to encompass a wider definition of health, e.g. to include psychosocial factors, probably makes it potentially more able to meet total health needs.

EVALUATING DOCTORS' DECISIONS

The methods of constraining clinical autonomy outlined above involve trying to control various input factors, whether informational or financial, in clinical decision making. The alternative is to persuade doctors to monitor their own work directly or to introduce more third-party evaluation of the results of those decisions.

CLINICAL AUDIT

Increasingly, doctors are being persuaded to introduce their own 'quality control' in clinical practice. This can take various forms, but essentially depends on doctors assessing some aspect of their performance against agreed standards of good-quality care. Any discrepancy between what does happen and what should happen is meant to lead to appropriate corrective action.

As long as doctors are willing to review the quality of their own work, the more likely they are to be able to keep the clinical autonomy that they so value; the alternative is to accept assessment by third parties such as managers and government.

PEER REVIEW

One means of preserving the principle of medical autonomy, yet enabling assessment of an individual doctor's work, is to introduce a peer review mechanism. In the USA, because of the dangers of over-operating as a result of the fee-for-service system, many hospitals have peer review committees to examine the pathology reports on surgically removed organs. If surgeons are over-operating, more histologically normal tissues are likely to be removed. This enables such surgeons to be identified and brought to task.

Britain has fewer peer review procedures, partly because over-treatment is not such a problem (except, perhaps, in the fee-for-service world of general dental practice). However, there is one form of peer review that deserves separate mention, and that is the Confidential Enquiry.

In the 1950s in Britain, a Confidential Enquiry was set up to examine the circumstances surrounding any woman's death during pregnancy and childbirth. The enquiry team is composed largely of professional members, and is required to take evidence from all concerned, reach a conclusion as to whether the death was preventable and, if so, who was to be held responsible.

Because the enquiry works confidentially, it is not a direct threat to clinical autonomy – even doctors who are held responsible in some way for a woman's death are not named. People are therefore happy to give evidence in the knowledge that the conclusions of the study might help improve procedures such that there would be no recurrence. In the event, maternal mortality has dropped sharply since the inception of the enquiry and, although it is impossible to say definitively whether the latter has been responsible, it is likely to have played some part. The idea of a confidential enquiry has now been extended to other areas of clinical practice, such as deaths following surgical operations, and provides a useful, non-threatening mechanism for ensuring high standards in areas of medicine in which the number of 'negative' events is relatively small (otherwise professionals could spend more time staffing enquiries than doing their clinical work!).

PERFORMANCE INDICATORS

In recent years, much management philosophy has moved towards performance indicators and performance-related pay. Choosing suitable indicators for clinical practice is difficult, but may be possible for some types of routine work. In many countries, mortality rates for hospitals – and even by surgeon – are being made public, though obviously there are many factors other than the quality of care (such as case severity) that lead to death. The idea of such indices is spreading, as health services struggle to ensure good-quality care with limited resources, though debates continue as to the real meaning of many indicators.

PATIENT ASSESSMENTS

Patients are in a position to comment on clinical decisions just as much as doctors and managers.

Satisfaction and complaints

To allow some redress against bad or inappropriate medical decisions, various complaints procedures have emerged. Some medical decisions are so mistaken that they go to litigation, but many are relatively minor, and only require the service to have some negative feedback to prevent the same thing happening again.

In the USA, patients complain and go to litigation with some enthusiasm. In Britain, with a long tradition of deference to medical authority, it has proved difficult to establish a fair and effective complaints machinery: very often it is hampered by constraints on the type of complaint that can be made, the time span after the incident in which it can be reported, the over-representation of doctors themselves on the adjudication panel, and the triviality of many penalties. Even so, whenever a complaint is made, doctors often find it a devastating experience.

There are two alternative strategies: one is to encourage more 'consumerism', in which patients are encouraged to change doctors, get second opinions, or go elsewhere if they do not get satisfaction; the other is to encourage the direct monitoring of patient satisfaction by means of surveys (DHSS 1987). Such surveys are becoming increasingly popular, though they can pose problems of measurement. Clearly, a patient's level of satisfaction with a service must reflect earlier expectations: high expectations are likely to lead to a more critical view, other things being equal (Locker and Dunt 1978). Also, it is often found that general levels of satisfaction with a service are higher than if more specific aspects of care are asked about (Williams and Calnan 1991).

Professional discipline

The medical profession has been given control over the content of its own work; but part of that 'contract' with society is that it will police its own members and discipline them as necessary. In the USA, this is the responsibility of the state medical disciplinary boards, which are dominated by the medical profession and have proved reluctant to discipline doctors for clinical incompetence other than that brought about by illness or frank criminal behaviour. The result is that Americans have turned to the law courts to obtain redress.

In Britain, the responsibility for disciplining doctors has also been controlled by doctors themselves, in this case through the General Medical Council (GMC). For many years, the GMC took little direct interest in questions of clinical competence and tended to concentrate on the five 'A's of alcoholism, advertising, addiction, adultery and abortion (though, since the legalization of abortion, the last less so). This has led to a growing willingness to seek legal recompense (as evidenced by increases in medical insurance premiums), though not to the extent of the USA, for reasons described below. A succession of 'scandals' involving incompetent clinicians has led the GMC to reform itself and – with some government encouragement – to introduce more rigorous procedures for assessing and disciplining doctors whose clinical skills are brought into question. Greater responsiveness to public concerns about standards in clinical care is likely to guide the profession's future; whether it can rely so much on self-regulation must be in some doubt (Rosenthal 1987).

Litigation

If all else fails, and the problem is sufficiently serious, patients have the right to pursue the medical profession for redress in court. In practice, this is a common strategy in the USA but relatively unusual in Britain.

First, it is probably fair to say that Americans are more litigious, being more prepared to use the law courts to obtain compensation (and often massive settlements if successful). Second, American lawyers make great use of the 'contingency fee' system, under which they are paid only if successful. This means that there is no financial risk for patients in going to court, and usually a generous percentage of any settlement for the winning lawyer. This has led to some lawyers deliberately seeking out dissatisfied patients to try to win a large sum in court. To pay for this system, medical insurance is very high – for high-risk specialties, several tens of thousands of dollars annually – leading to compensatory higher clinical fees in these areas.

American court settlements can be extraordinarily high and there is continuing doubt as to whether the increasing costs can be carried by doctors and hospitals. One solution being mooted is to separate compensation from the issue of whether the doctor has been negligent by setting up a no-fault insurance plan that would compensate patients whatever the cause of their problem (Rosenthal 1987). This still leaves the need for a strengthened medical disciplinary procedure to identify and deal with those incompetent doctors whose actions can be so harmful to their patients.

CLINICAL GOVERNANCE

An important way of thinking about the tension between exercising some control over clinical decisions while allowing doctors some freedom to act in the interests of their patients is to see the problem in terms of clinical governance: in other words, how is clinical work to be 'governed'?. In the past, the control of clinical work has almost gone by default: the individual practitioner could be relied upon to act responsibly. For many of the reasons outlined above, this informal system failed. Governance must now be taken more seriously. How exactly should and how can doctors be governed?

An important principle of clinical governance is that it is best exercised by doctors themselves. The shift, however, is to make it the responsibility of the collective rather than of the individual. In other words, doctors as a group must take responsibility for the clinical behaviour of individual doctors. For example, a hospital might appoint a clinician to lead on clinical governance in that hospital. That person will then discuss with colleagues the sorts of actions they should take collectively to ensure that good-quality care is being provided. It may mean stricter adherence to protocols, or expectations that all clinicians will engage in auditing their own work, or arranging for peer review of certain services, or setting up a complaints system, or monitoring of prescribing etc. The result is a culture of quality control in which all clinicians are aware that they are part of a wider attempt to maintain medical standards through reviewing their own as well as their colleagues' clinical performance.

Chapter 12

ORGANIZING HEALTH CARE

Although health care is found in all countries, there is a variety of ways in which it is organized. Broadly, these range from a market system, in which health care is treated as any other private commodity, to that of universal free entitlement underwritten by government funding. The particular form of health care in a country reflects both its history and current political philosophy, the market system being more likely to be supported by the political right and government provision by the left. As governments grapple with increasing demands for health care – together with ever-rising costs – the differences between the political right and left is becoming less distinct, as all face common problems.

ALLOCATING SCARCE RESOURCES

Health care, as any economic system of production and distribution, starts with the assumption of scarce resources. This means that there are not enough resources – in this case health care – to enable everyone to consume what they would like. It follows that there needs to be a mechanism for distributing these scarce resources in some way. This mechanism is often referred to as 'rationing'. Rationing has unhappy echoes of wartime deprivation and there are those who claim that health care is too important to be rationed. Nevertheless, the amount of health care that could be consumed by all citizens is virtually infinite: just imagine everyone using daily psychotherapy after a busy day, or perhaps some form of physiotherapy to help them relax. Of course, in these circumstances some health care would be judged a waste of resources, but, equally, in a very basic health care system, some less than rudimentary health care might be judged indulgent for that system. In short, all health care systems are about rationing health care (though the rationing might not be obvious) and, even if resources were increased, this would change the level of rationing but not the need to continue to ration. Sometimes 'resource priorities' and 'resource allocation' are viewed as more politically acceptable terms than rationing, but the underlying need to choose between alternatives remains.

THE MARKET SYSTEM

The solution of the market economy to the problem of scarce resources is to allow individual consumers to make choices about how they will spend their incomes.

As incomes are limited, consumers must choose between alternatives: buying a car, perhaps, or a holiday, or a surgical operation. Taken together, these different consumer choices focus attention on shortages in the economy: if there is greater demand for cars than for holidays, productive resources will move from providing holidays into car production. The mechanism for this movement is the 'profit motive', as producers see there is more money to be made from making cars than providing holidays. In addition, because of the demand for cars, it would be expected that the salaries available in the car industry would be greater than those available in the holiday industry, in which case people would change jobs and gradually move into those parts of the economy that were expanding to meet consumer demand.

In practice, of course, major shifts in salaries do not occur, as there are various mechanisms in Western societies that prevent such radical changes (these are constraints that economists say make the market 'inefficient'). However, consumer choice and efficient shifts in production in response to that choice remain essential characteristics of the market economy.

An important feature of the market economy is that consumption is determined by disposable income and consumer choices. This may be a simple fact of life when considering the purchase of a car (not enough money to buy the model you want, or even to buy a car at all?), but becomes a major problem when vital health care is needed but the person does not have the income to buy it. For example, although the USA spends more than any other country on health care, the fact that it has relied largely on market mechanisms for its distribution/rationing means that there are many people who are deprived of what others would consider essential health care through their inability to purchase the required service. But which government can tolerate people dying through lack of basic care when resources are potentially available? The failure to provide care for a proportion of the population because it lacks the income to access the service has proved politically unacceptable, and alternative rationing mechanisms have been introduced to compensate.

THE COMMAND SYSTEM

The other way of organizing the production and distribution of resources in a society is the command or directed economy. In this system, people's needs are determined by central authorities. In other words, it is not what consumers wish or demand that affects what they consume, but rather what they 'need'. Once all needs have been determined, production is organized to meet those needs, with goods and services allocated accordingly.

This system can go hopelessly wrong and can be remarkably inefficient. Former economies in Eastern Europe were renowned for deciding that their populations needed so many pairs of shoes per year, producing those shoes, then finding that the population chose not to buy them. The principle, however, is an important one: that the function of an economic system is to meet people's needs rather than their more capricious wishes, which are, in their turn, dependent on having the resources to satisfy them.

An example of the central government deciding to 'ration' a resource rather than allow the market to buy and sell on the basis of price is the right to vote: all adult citizens are given one vote irrespective of their income or wealth. Another example is government provision of education for all children: the government decides that all citizens need a level of basic education whatever their individual preferences. Some parents might choose to send their child to a private school, but they still have the right to use state-provided education. In similar fashion, choosing to view health care as a right, just like the right to vote or to receive schooling, means that governments must provide at least the basics of a health care system for all citizens.

The major differences between market and command economic systems are shown in Table 12.1.

Table 12.1 Differences between market and state provision of health care

	Market	**State provision**
Health care	A commodity	A right
Consumer options	Wishes/choice	Needs/no choice
Resource	'Invisible hand'	Explicit rationing
Allocation	Efficient	'Inefficient'
Access	Unequal	Equity
Social justice	Unfair to many	Fair

For the market economy, health care is treated as a commodity. This means that while people have a choice – whether to buy it or not – some people will find that they do not have the resources to buy the amount they feel they need. The command economy, on the other hand, treats health care as a right of all citizens. In this case, government provision ensures equity – that is, to each according to his or her health needs.

Health care provision in all countries seems to be constantly in a state of flux. No country seems to get it perfectly right. The reason for this is that an ideal health care system would probably take the idea of choice together with the efficiency of resource allocation from the market system, and the meeting of all health needs from the command system. The paradox is that as choice/efficiency is increased, so the level of equity usually declines, and vice versa.

THE INSURANCE PRINCIPLE

Unlike most other consumer goods and services, health care needs are unpredictable, meaning that large expenses can accrue quickly and unexpectedly. Thus, whereas expenditure on items such as transport, housing, food etc. can be fairly reliably predicted and therefore budgeted for, health expenditure for an individual can be almost non-existent one year, then sudden and large the next.

The usual strategy for dealing with unpredictable and costly risks is insurance.

Few people are willing to risk the cost of rebuilding their house after a major fire or replacing their car after a serious accident; they therefore take out insurance. This means, in effect, that all people taking out insurance spread the cost of replacing the relatively few damaged cars or houses when they occur. Exactly the same principle applies to health care. All the people who take out insurance spread the risk and therefore the cost of paying for expensive medical bills. Insurance therefore provides a mechanism for people to access health care within a market system that would otherwise demand large, if infrequent, payments.

One way to pay for health care is to take out insurance with a third-party insurance company. In effect, the insurance company acts as intermediary between the patient and the health care marketplace. Health insurance can be arranged privately or through an employer's scheme, often with the employer paying or contributing to the premiums. The insurer agrees to meet the costs of health care needed by the patient. The patient then visits doctors or hospitals, is charged a fee for the services rendered, and then either the patient or the doctor reclaims the money from the insurance body.

In many countries, health insurance is compulsory, in that contributions are deducted from pay packets alongside income tax. Employers are often required to make a matching contribution. However, this method of paying for health care is only open to those in employment, and other mechanisms of ensuring health care is available have to be established for those not covered.

Whereas the insurance principle enables the consumer to deal with the unexpected nature and high cost of health care, the principle does undermine the central market discipline that consumers have limited resources and therefore must choose between competing demands. This problem is magnified by a key difference between health care demands and claims made under other insurance policies such as those that cover a car or house. In the latter, there is both an upper limit on the claim – presumably the cost of replacement – and a general agreement of what counts as a legitimate claim. In health care, however, especially with new and expensive treatments, there might be no clear 'maximum' claim and little agreement on what is really needed in a particular case. In effect, having taken out insurance, consumers are able to consume health services with few real constraints. The net effect of this situation has been steeply rising costs of health care.

In an attempt to bring this situation under some sort of control in recent years, insurers have tried to limit costs in the following ways.

- By shifting some of the costs back on to the consumer to act as a disincentive to further use. Patients might be required to pay for certain specific services or a percentage of the cost of others. Faced with such costs, consumers might be persuaded to limit their demands. However, this strategy is only of limited scope, as the whole principle of insurance is to remove the threat of significant immediate direct costs.
- By limiting the amount of payment to doctors and hospitals on the basis of the patient's particular medical problem. Diagnosis-related groups (DRGs: see

Chapter 11) encourage both doctor and hospital to restrain their expenditure to the expected amount they will receive.

- By meeting the consumer's health needs but limiting choice to certain cost-contained health services, as in Health Maintenance Organizations (HMOs).

HMOs have proved very popular in the USA in recent years. Patients pay a regular insurance premium and get access to primary care physicians in the HMO (often paid by capitation or salary), who then, if necessary, refer them to hospitals either owned or contracted to the HMO. Patient choice is therefore severely curtailed and costs are tightly controlled, both at the level of primary care and in the payments made to hospitals.

The financial success of HMOs can be gauged by the fact that they turn out to be 10–40 per cent cheaper than traditional fee-for-service medical practice. Their success seems to be mainly in keeping patients out of hospital – which is the most expensive part of health care. In addition, in having mainly salaried doctors, there is no incentive for doctors to over-treat. Doctors employed by HMOs are also closely monitored in terms of their work patterns and workload.

It has been claimed that the salaried doctors who are attracted to HMOs are those doctors who are unable to make a living in the usual fee-for-service environment. Critics of HMOs therefore argue that HMO doctors tend to be clinically less able – or, more charitably, it might be that they are less business-like. The suspicion that they are less competent, coupled with the fact that their salaried status leads them to under-treat rather than over-treat and that there are financial limits on the care that will be provided, has led to a belief in the USA that the quality of care given by HMOs is lower than that given by traditional private fee-for-service medicine.

Also, just as hospitals that are operating with DRGs may carefully select the sorts of patients they treat, so HMOs have a financial incentive to enrol only patients who are healthy. Elderly patients, patients with chronic illness etc. may therefore find it difficult to join an HMO.

The third practical difficulty of HMOs is arranging health cover when patients are outside the area. A patient taken ill on holiday or requiring urgent accident and emergency treatment can reclaim the costs from their HMO, but only within very strict guidelines.

Insurance-based health care, as in HMOs, is meant to provide the traditional market benefit of choice, but the need to contain costs has meant it has been inexorably worn away. However, a more fundamental problem with relying on insurance to access the marketplace is that it only partly addresses the underlying problem of people being denied adequate health care. For many, a relatively small monthly premium covers potential medical problems in the future; but others choose to take a risk that they will not get ill and/or need expensive health care. For some this gamble will work, but others will be caught with health care needs and inadequate resources. Perhaps they should pay the price of their failed gamble – but it is then difficult to refuse them health care.

More commonly, the problem is not that patients have lost the gamble that they would not get ill, but that they do not have the resources to pay the initial health insurance premiums. The response to this problem has been government intervention to provide a sort of safety net for those too poor to obtain any health care. In addition, many people who take out insurance only buy a limited policy, which may not provide sufficient cover for the expenses of a catastrophic illness. The net effect of this is that patients faced with large medical bills first use their insurance cover to pay them, as far as it will go; next they pay with their own money – this may involve them selling all their material assets; then, when they are virtually destitute, they will qualify for government support. For this reason, the largest cause of individual bankruptcy in the USA is health care costs. (In practice, some of these bankruptcies are only technical, in that some people arrange their financial affairs so as to appear poor enough to qualify for government support when large medical bills are seen as imminent.)

The fact that it is seen as politically and socially unacceptable to deprive people of basic health care – even though the market system would argue that some people should go without health care, just as some people go without a car – means that all governments have been drawn into providing, at the very least, a sort of insurance cover of last resort to their populations. In the USA, this has taken the form of Medicare for old people and Medicaid for the very poor. These schemes represent a sort of compulsory, subsidized insurance through government. In Continental Europe, such arrangements – covering most if not all of the population – are popular.

GOVERNMENT INTERVENTION IN HEALTH CARE

In Britain, private practice has always played a part for those patients affluent enough to buy health care directly, but in the past the poor could only rely on services based on charity, traditionally through the church, then, from the eighteenth century, through philanthropy. During the nineteenth century, the insurance principle began to govern more of health care provision as groups of workers found they could contribute a small weekly premium to a non-profit-making Friendly Society and obtain cover for general practitioner (GP) services. However, welfare systems based on these principles could not succeed in meeting the health care needs of all the population, and the government has been gradually drawn into providing care – at first through a sort of safety net for those who slipped through the other systems, and later on a more comprehensive basis.

Government intervention in welfare can be traced back to the Elizabethan Poor Laws, which set up workhouses for the destitute. As poverty and illness have always been closely related, it was not long before workhouses were looking after the chronically sick. By the twentieth century, (local) government found itself the direct funding source for many hospitals that had emerged from the old workhouse system. In 1948, with the introduction of the National Health Service (NHS), central government took over the locally controlled hospitals and brought into public ownership the acute hospitals based on the old system of charity, thereby becoming the paymaster for almost all hospital provision in Britain.

The government had also been drawn into organizing primary health care early in the twentieth century, when it took over and extended the role of Friendly Societies by introducing a National Health Insurance scheme for GP services. Insurance premiums were paid to the government in the form of deductions from pay packets; these premiums then funded general practice cover for that person and their family. This system was extended to all the population in 1948 with the advent of the NHS. Some funding continued from National Health Insurance charges on wages and salaries, but the overall cost of the health service far exceeded these insurance premiums and very rapidly came to rely on revenues raised through general taxation for the bulk of its expenditure. In effect, in 1948 in Britain the government moved from being the organizer of the insurance system to being the direct provider of services for all citizens as a civic right. The NHS therefore became a major example of a health care system based not on the market but on the command system of resource allocation.

From the inception of the NHS in 1948, the political philosophy behind health care provision in Britain has been equity – that is, the provision of health care should be on the basis of need. Health care should not therefore be given to people because they have high status, power or wealth, but because they need the care. In the main, doctors are paid by salary and capitation, so they have no incentive to assign health services other than on the basis of need.

PROBLEMS OF GOVERNMENT-FUNDED HEALTH CARE PROVISION

From its inception, the NHS faced a number of major problems.

- The major problem with a system of health care based on a principle of equity was that someone needed to define need. Who should do this? Doctors? Politicians? Managers?
- A related problem was the explicit need to ration services. In the market system, services are rationed by the ability of people to pay. Because no payment is made in a wholly government-provided system (which is free at the point of delivery), there have to be other rationing mechanisms that may be politically unpopular.
- Because health need was not defined by the patient, the system tended to be paternalistic and took little heed of consumer preferences.
- The system was said to be inefficient in the way it allocated resources, because it was unresponsive to rapid changes in health care needs.

IMPROVING CHOICE AND EFFICIENCY

Some of the above problems were dealt with by permitting, and indeed encouraging, a private sector for health care delivery. This enabled patients to have choice within the private sector and choice between the private and public sectors (with the proviso, of course, that only those with resources were able to make these choices). In addition, a number of attempts were made to influence the way the NHS provided its services.

- Improvements in administrative coherence and management efficiency: this was tackled either by re-organizing the administrative structure of the health service or by introducing professional managers into health care delivery to ensure efficient use of resources.
- Increasing constraints on clinical autonomy, which traditionally enabled doctors to define need and dispense resources (see Chapter 11).
- Government intervention to try to make resource allocation as rational as possible: this meant that funds were allocated to different regions of the health service on the basis of their population and health care need.
- Introduction of competition into the various NHS services, such as catering and laundry, by inviting tenders from private companies to provide the service.

Despite these measures, there were still complaints about the way the NHS worked and about the lack of sufficient funding. The government was eventually forced to set up a review of how the NHS was organized, and the outcome of this process was a major reform of the NHS (Department of Health 1989). Instead of providing a major new influx of resources, the government decided that the way forward was to make existing public funding work more efficiently by introducing market mechanisms in an attempt to improve efficiency.

MANAGED COMPETITION

Despite the success of a directly government-funded 'universal' health care service in providing an equitable system of health care delivery, problems remained. In particular:

- *Rising costs*. In 1948, there was a belief that the success of the British NHS would decrease the amount of illness in the community so that its costs would decline. This was very much mistaken: costs have risen several-fold in real terms (that is, allowing for inflation). Health care has become a major cost to central government.
- *Inefficiency*. A related issue was the perceived inefficiency of a system that had no incentives to maximize value for money. In the market system, efficiency emerges from the competition between providers, who are forced to reduce their prices and improve efficiency if they are to survive. In a government-funded health service, there was no need for hospitals or doctors to examine how efficient they were, as funding continued from year to year irrespective of the value for money that they offered.
- *Unresponsiveness*. Consumer feedback is an important market mechanism. If consumers do not like the price or quality of any goods or services, in future they will shop elsewhere. However, in a rather paternalistic government-

funded service, consumers, in the form of patients, were given little choice in the care they received and the NHS took little interest in consumer feedback, as it seemed to have little relevance to its goal of providing a good basic level of care to everyone. However, the consumerist revolution of the late twentieth century did not leave health services untouched. Why should patients accept a second-rate service and be expected to be grateful for whatever care they received? Patients' satisfaction is itself gradually became an increasingly important marker of clinical success (see Chapter 11). Moreover, by harnessing patients' views, perhaps the overall efficiency of the service might be improved.

In summary, the critic could argue that once government funding appeared in large amounts, providers began to lose any incentive to remain efficient and patients were increasingly given care predetermined by a government bureaucracy that administered the purse strings. The solution seemed to be something that combined the best of public and private, and this emerged in the ideas of 'managed competition' and 'internal markets' (Light 2001).

The essence of health service reforms introduced into the British NHS and mooted in the USA is to separate the funding of health services from their supply. For reasons described above, governments feel an obligation to ensure that all citizens have access to health care; therefore, they must provide the necessary funding for that care. However, rather than give the money directly to hospitals, doctors etc., they have set up a competitive environment in health care by requiring providers to compete against one another for the available resources. This has been achieved by giving the money to an intermediate body of health service 'purchasers', who are charged with obtaining the best value for the people they have in their jurisdiction. The amount of money given to these purchasers (or commissioners of health care, as they are often known) is based on a fixed sum for everyone living in the particular area. Then, with this money, the purchasers negotiate with health care providers (mainly hospitals) to obtain the best care deals for the money available.

THE INTERNAL MARKET

GPs have a dual role in the new system in the NHS. On the one hand, they are providers of (primary) health care to their populations; but, on the other, they act as the purchasers of secondary care for their patients. Groups of GPs are given funds to cover the secondary care they are likely to need for their patients. They then negotiate with hospital providers to arrange appropriate contracts. In effect, a quasi-marketplace is set up between consumers and providers of health care. However, instead of consumers negotiating with providers, they rely on a third party, the purchasers, to do it on their behalf; this ensures that individual needs/wants are balanced within existing resource constraints. Providers for their part are placed in a more market-orientated environment, though one with purchasers rather than consumers to please.

This system embodies some of the advantages of the market in that health care providers, particularly in the form of hospitals, must compete against each other to obtain contracts to provide services for the purchaser's population. Moreover, the purchaser is in a position to try to assess the needs of the local population and purchase services appropriately. In the past, the particular service provided was determined largely by the providers, usually dominated by hospital doctors' opinions. Arguably, some of these choices of services reflected more on doctors' pet areas of interest and medical fashion than on a dispassionate assessment of how all health care resources might best be deployed to obtain maximum health gain for the population. In the new system, health providers must bid against one another to provide services that the purchasers have determined represent the best options for their local population.

Despite the appeal of the new arrangements – services that reflect patients' needs and obtained at the best price – there are certain practical problems with the new system.

- To succeed, an internal market requires a number of competing health care providers. However, for many services, competition is limited. In some areas of the country there may be only one hospital serving the local population, and even when there is more than one, some services, for example accident and emergency, might be dictated by the need for rapid local access rather than by who can provide the cheapest price.
- Purchasers reach agreement with providers by means of contracts between them. However, contracts are very difficult to specify. For certain well-defined procedures such as hip replacement, it is relatively easy to purchase, say, 200 per annum. But for a non-specific emergency admission, the cost implications can vary between a small amount for a few antibiotics to major and expensive transplant surgery.
- The ideal of the market is that it gives consumers the power to make their own choices. However, despite the importance of 'consumerism' in motivating recent health care reforms, it is ironic that a system of purchasers/providers almost completely excludes the actual consumers of care. In effect, the decisions to purchase or not are being made on the consumers' behalf by the new purchasing managers. (Of course, consumers could not be allowed to make these decisions: if they relied on the same defined pool of resources for buying those services, there is no way to prevent them buying more services than the resources permit. Equally, giving resources to individuals to spend either in the form of cash or vouchers ignores the fact that some consumers of health care have much greater needs than others.)
- The market is 'efficient' because it drives down prices through competition. One inevitable consequence of this process is that inefficient producers are driven out of business. If the same logic were applied to health care, there should be some hospitals going bankrupt. Whether this is politically acceptable is another matter, especially if the hospital provides essential services to a local community.

Still, despite these problems, the separation into purchasing and providing functions does cause a reassessment of the way health has traditionally been provided. Somewhat ironically in view of the stress on the importance of local markets, there is now a greater central control over health service priorities. Purchasers can look at the total health needs of their populations and buy services in the light of these. Some services, such as tattoo removal or infertility treatments, are not purchased (on the grounds that they are not appropriate for a health care service or they are expensive and/or have a poor success rate). Also, although contracts are not very specific or sensitive, it is still possible to build in 'quality' indicators such as acceptable waiting times and a requirement to carry out regular audits of services.

For providers, there is a real incentive to ensure that only cost-effective treatments are used. For both purchasers and providers, there is now a freedom to innovate – to think creatively about the optimal care that can be provided, whether this is a greater emphasis on day surgery or bringing in osteopaths to treat backache. The new thinking extends to blurring the distinction between private and public supply of services. A hospital can bid for a contract irrespective of whether it is in the public domain or not – the task of the purchasers is simply to secure the best-quality services at the best price, wherever they might be found. As a corollary, previously directly funded NHS hospitals now have the option of greater financial independence (as Trust hospitals) and more freedom to make local management decisions.

THE FUTURE OF HEALTH CARE

It is apparent from the collapse of command economies in Eastern Europe that market economics has triumphed. This belief in the power of markets has now been seen in reforms of Western health care systems, including the NHS. To a large extent, these reforms have meant a culture shock for systems long grown used to regular direct government support, and a challenge to become more efficient.

Even so, use of the market as a mechanism for distributing resources is compromised by the way it is easily distorted and abused. Health care in the future is therefore likely, on the one hand, to promote the success of market mechanisms and, on the other hand, to restrain potential abuses.

In the USA, there are regular moves to improve the operation of the health care market. For example, the monopoly position of health care providers, particularly doctors, is a serious impediment to the market, and successive US governments have tried to oppose such monopolies by encouraging advertising, liberalizing entry into medicine etc. In addition, the patients' position in the market can be strengthened by improving patient knowledge (the idea of fully informed consent) and by enabling litigation to proceed when consumers are dissatisfied. The internet also provides consumers with enormous amounts of new information about health, illness and health care, enabling them more easily to challenge professional claims to expertise.

Yet, for all their virtues, 'free' markets still need some sort of regulation, otherwise the freedom is exploited, particularly by producers who form cartels to fix prices and sell shoddy goods and services to an unsuspecting public. Thus health care markets need their own regulatory mechanisms to prevent abuses, just as the insurance market requires that insurance agents are registered and follow a code of practice, and the fruit and vegetable market is subject to regular inspection of weighing scales. One solution is to lay down centrally determined 'quality-control' criteria – dictating which treatments can and cannot be used, setting out optimal disease management patterns (as in managed care), regular inspection of facilities etc. The problem is that central control and regulations will begin to stifle the energy that markets undoubtedly release, as well as much of the discretion that individual doctors might feel they need to practise in the patients' best interests. In a sense, all health services must try to achieve a balance between centrally determined 'rules' that enforce best practice on otherwise idiosyncratic local practices and allowing individuals to show initiative so that on-the-ground judgements can be made about what is best for individual patients.

The key message for the organization of health care is that there is no ideal system, no panacea that will deliver everything. All health care provision is a compromise between different philosophies in an attempt to obtain the best of all worlds. At the moment, the market is in the ascendancy, as 'managed competition'' is the international flavour, but the debate is far from over (Glaser 1993).

Finally, does the organization of health care matter? Never mind the politics; what is the actual effect on health of different ways of organizing health care? First, the question needs to be placed in context. Variation in public spending across different countries (no matter how health care is organized) explains less than one-seventh of 1 per cent of observed differences in mortality across those countries. On the other hand, 95 per cent of cross-sectional variation in mortality can be explained by a country's income per capita, inequality of income distribution, extent of female education, level of ethnic fragmentation and predominant religion (Filmer and Pritchett 1999). This puts into clearer perspective the role of health care relative to the importance of these other social factors. If overall health care expenditure plays such a small part in the big picture, it is unlikely that different ways of organizing health care will have dramatic effects on a nation's health. Ironically, it may be in its relationship with these other, more important, factors, such as inequality, that the organization of health care can make its strongest claim to matter.

Chapter 13

EVALUATING HEALTH CARE

What are the costs and benefits of consuming health care? Four different questions can be asked.

1 Is health care effective/efficient?
2 Does it meet 'real' needs?
3 Is it fair?
4 Is it iatrogenic?

IS HEALTH CARE EFFECTIVE/EFFICIENT?

It is obvious that health care should be effective, otherwise it represents a waste of resources.

EFFECTIVENESS

To evaluate the effectiveness of a particular medical intervention, it is necessary to compare the initial state with the result or outcome of treatment. However, an improvement does not necessarily imply that the intervention was effective, because the natural course of the health problem may have produced exactly the same improvement. For example, if the common cold were to be treated with antibiotics, it would be found that all patients were cured. However, the reason they were cured was not the antibiotics (which are ineffective against viruses), but the natural course of the infection.

In any evaluation it is therefore important to allow for other influences, particularly natural progression, on the outcome. The way around this problem was discovered several decades ago when the *randomized controlled clinical trial* (RCT) came into use. Patients for whom a certain treatment may be of benefit are randomly allocated to an intervention and a control group. The purpose of randomization is to distribute all other factors, known and unknown, that might affect outcome evenly between both groups so that any difference in outcome must be due to the intervention. The intervention group receives the treatment (preferably 'blind'), the control group receives a placebo (or alternative treatment), and the outcomes in the two groups are then compared. If the results in the intervention group are better than the results in the control group, it can then be said that the treatment is effective; on the other hand, if outcomes are similar in both groups, the treatment is ineffective (or no better than the existing treatment against which it was compared).

It has been claimed that use of these techniques would enable the objective assessment of medical treatments (Cochrane 1972). Nevertheless, it has been estimated that less than 20 per cent of all medical interventions have been properly evaluated for their effectiveness. Medicine continues to rely on 'tried and tested' interventions that have not been shown to be effective or – and in some ways more important – shown to be safe. Arguably, a lot more can be done to test and improve the effectiveness of medical interventions. This view has led to the development of 'evidence-based medicine' that prioritizes the rigorous scrutiny and collation of evidence on different investigations and treatments.

Evidence-based medicine involves a way of thinking critically about different aspects of clinical practice. First, it makes the RCT the gold standard of clinical effectiveness: if a well-designed RCT shows that some treatment works (or does not work), this evidence would be more persuasive than any other. In effect, there is a hierarchy of evidence from the RCT at the pinnacle through studies without randomization but with control groups to simple descriptions at the base. Second, it recognizes that evidence accumulates and techniques are needed to collate it all together. Two important techniques are meta-analysis, which combines the results of many inconclusive trials to generate a more precise understanding of the treatment, and systematic reviews, which attempt by rigorous selection and analysis of papers to draw the most valid conclusion about whether or not a certain treatment works.

Evidence-based medicine has been very successful at identifying and promoting effective treatments. It has been less successful at persuading clinicians to endorse wholeheartedly and use these effective treatments; Chapter 11 outlines some of the difficulties in involving doctors in policies that may constrain their clinical autonomy.

No doubt randomized controlled trials are immensely important in examining the effectiveness of treatments, but they are not always possible, and their results often need treating with some caution.

- Sometimes ethical considerations prevent patients from being randomized to a potentially harmful group (usually claimed to be the placebo group).
- Results from a trial may be limited by the size and type of population that is randomized; thus, sometimes two different trials produce contrary results.
- Trials usually compare treatments on one parameter, sometimes deaths or other biological measures. But, of course, it is possible that one treatment may produce a certain type of improvement – say, increased life expectancy – whereas another might improve some factors – such as quality of life. The choice is then between two treatments that are successful in different ways.
- Trials produce evidence in terms of the 'number needed to treat' (NNT) – that is, how many patients need to be treated for one to benefit. The Medical Research Council (MRC) trial of treatment of mild hypertension, for example,

found that lowering blood pressure did work, but that 850 patients needed to be treated for a year for one patient to avoid a non-fatal stroke. This finding then needs to be translated into clinical policy: should mild hypertension be treated and who should decide (Misselbrook and Armstrong 2001)?

RATIONING

Even accepting that one treatment is better than another, does this justify its use for a patient who would benefit from it? Given that the resources of a health service are finite, by providing one patient with an effective therapy for a problem, another patient is deprived of those same resources. If renal dialysis is provided for a patient, the cost of that treatment is not then available to provide care for a geriatric patient, or an improved antenatal service, or radiotherapy for a cancer. All health care, whether implicitly or explicitly, involves some sort of rationing (Aaron and Schwartz 1984).

Limited health care resources (and they always are limited in some way) mean that the doctor's decision to help one patient is, paradoxically, depriving another patient. Thus, although doctors are taught to treat individual patients to the best of their ability, and though they may be wise enough only to use effective methods, they are, in fact, constantly making non-individual judgements; their decision to treat one patient is also a decision to allocate resources away from other potential patients the doctor probably has not even seen or may not know about. Every treatment is, in effect, a judgement on health care priorities.

EFFICIENCY

Because all health care systems work with scarce resources, it is important that health care is efficient. Efficiency means that maximum benefit is obtained for each unit of resources. Two drugs might be equally effective at treating a patient, but if one costs twice as much as the other, then the more efficient treatment is the cheaper one. Similarly, although medical advice to give up smoking is relatively ineffective (only a few per cent of patients will respond), the fact that it is a very cheap therapy – only a few minutes of a doctor's time – means that it is probably a very efficient treatment compared with, say, renal dialysis, even though the latter is much more effective.

Given the importance of not only knowing whether a medical intervention works but also whether it is a reasonable procedure to provide for patients in terms of its cost, health economists have devised a number of different ways of examining the relative costs and benefits of health care.

Cost minimization analysis

This is the simplest technique, but depends on having two treatments that have very similar results. In such circumstances, it would seem logical to choose the cheaper treatment so as to minimize costs. For example, if aspirin and an expensive non-steroidal anti-inflammatory drug (NSAID) both have the same effect on a patient's arthritic pain, it would be appropriate to choose the cheaper aspirin.

Cost–benefit analysis

Cost–benefit analysis compares the outcomes of treatments in monetary terms. For example, a drug that enabled a patient to be returned to work earlier than another could be valued in terms of the financial benefits of such an outcome. It is then a relatively easy task to compare the cost of the drugs with the financial benefits they produce so as to choose the best-value treatment.

Cost-effectiveness analysis

Sometimes one treatment is found to be better than another but also more expensive. A cost-effectiveness analysis is appropriate here to establish whether the extra cost is worth it in terms of benefit for the patient. Cost-effectiveness requires that the same measure of effect is used to compare interventions. This means that treatments can then be compared in terms of cost per unit of effect achieved, e.g. cost per extra year of life lived, or cost per decrease in millimetres of diastolic blood pressure.

Cost–utility analysis

A major problem with cost-effectiveness studies is that treatments are compared in terms of one common effect. However, medical intervention often produces a number of different effects and, if these are to be compared, there needs to be a way of reducing them to a common 'currency'. This can be achieved by asking people to weight their preferences for different outcomes and add the results. For example, someone may value being pain free as twice as important as being breathless. These weights reflect people's preferences and in economic jargon are called utilities – hence cost–utility analysis.

Cost-utility studies are becoming more common as it becomes necessary to make difficult choices about what can be afforded in health care provision. An example of a utility measure is a 'quality-adjusted life year' (QALY), as it attempts to combine a number of different facets of outcome into one number.

Essentially, a QALY involves identifying the costs of a number of different treatments and comparing these with extra years of life expectancy achieved, correcting for the quality of life during these extra years (presumably 2 years of life of a high quality would be preferred to 3 years of very poor quality). The calculation needs:

- a health status measure,
- the number of years of life expectancy,
- a discount rate.

There are a number of different ways of establishing a suitable health status measure – all based on obtaining the opinions of a range of people to act as a sort of benchmark. One is to use a 'standard gamble': what risks would people take on being fully healthy or dying for a given condition. This has proved difficult to implement, and other researchers have explored 'time trade-off'. Time trade-off requires subjects to find equivalent balances of illness severity against time. Thus, people would find it preferable to have full health over a certain time period, but, if they could live over a longer time period, what impairment of health would they be prepared to accept? These health–time combinations can then be adjusted so that subjects value them all equally; this then allows a value to be placed on a certain illness state. Alternatively, using discrete-choice modelling, respondents can be asked to express preferences between pairs of options – 'Would you like the operation to be within 2 months or would you rather wait for a surgeon of your choice?' – and these various preferences can then be used to 'model' the relative importance that people place on certain aspects of their care.

Another approach is to obtain evaluations of various illness states in terms of different degrees of distress (from none to severe) and disability (from none to unconscious). By getting a group of people to value different combinations of distress and disability, it is possible to give each a numerical score. Then, when a certain illness is placed in the distress–disability matrix, the appropriate score can be read off. Of course, with all of these techniques the values placed on illnesses are determined by the standards established by the study respondents, and these have often not been very representative of the whole population. But, then, whose values should define the standard? Different people would be expected to have different values depending on their age, gender, social background etc., and ill people themselves are likely to put values on being healthy that are very different values from those of people without illness.

The number of years of increased life expectancy for a certain condition is obtained from trials of the treatments. The calculation is rounded off with a 'discount rate'. This is an economist's way of saying that years of life in the future are worth less than years of life now. The principle seems a fair one, but the problem is that the discount rate selected (2 per cent? 5 per cent? 10 per cent?) can significantly affect the results of the calculation.

An example of some QALYs is given in Table 13.1. In examining this table, it is important to be aware that numbers such as these have been derived from a great number of different sources, often with very different underlying assumptions (Mason et al. 1993). Nevertheless, QALYs illustrate in a clear way that it is becoming increasingly important to compare value for money in all aspects of health provision.

Table 13.1 Quality-adjusted life years (QALYs) of competing therapies

	Cost per QALY (August 1990)
GP advice to stop smoking	270
Hip replacement	1 180
Kidney transplant	4 710
Breast cancer screening	5 780
Home dialysis	17 260
Hospital dialysis	21 970

DOES THE HEALTH CARE SYSTEM MEET THE 'REAL' NEEDS OF ITS CONSUMERS?

THE ROLE OF MEDICINE

Before it is possible to decide whether health care is successful in meeting the needs of its population, there must be some agreement as to what those needs really are. To many people, a legitimate goal of health care might be to save lives. However, the evidence presented in Chapter 4 would suggest that, over the years, medicine has not been very successful at this task. Indeed, although therapeutic value might be the chief rationale for a health service, it is clear from the problems of measurement (see Chapter 3) that this is difficult to quantify, as many factors other than the existence of health care seem to affect outcomes. Using the arguments advanced in Chapter 4 on the influence of social factors on morbidity and mortality, it might be argued that the specific therapeutic effect of a health service is fairly low in terms of lives saved or people cured – housing or diet, for example, may have a greater influence.

Yet to evaluate medicine by mortality would be a needless restriction. Indeed, the failure of medicine to make a marked impression on mortality led McKeown to argue that the role of medicine was wider than increasing life expectancy (1979). He suggested that medicine had four important roles:

1 to assist us to come safely into the world,
2 to support us comfortably out of the world,
3 to protect the healthy,
4 to care for the sick and disabled.

Although these goals may be less glamorous than those of curative medicine, they may be no less socially desirable. Also, whereas they too present considerable measurement problems (what is good care?), it is apparent that, in the context of the huge demands for health care, they probably represent important outcome criteria.

A TYPOLOGY OF NEED

Bradshaw (1972) suggested that need can be defined in four different ways.

1 *Felt need* refers to the perceptions of patients when they feel ill.
2 *Expressed need* describes the process by which felt need gets translated into demands on health services. Illness behaviour (see Chapter 2) is the framework in which patients express these needs.
3 *Normative need* refers to the definition of need by professionals – doctors, nurses, social workers etc.
4 *Comparative need* is used to compare two or more patients or populations. It sidesteps the question of whether this patient or population has a real need by exploring the extent to which it has a need relative to another patient or population.

All four types of need are to be found in health care. Patients' views of need – felt and expressed – are addressed in models of illness that emphasize the importance of patients' own views for their health status. However, patient definitions of need also appear in demands for health care, whether expressed directly, as in requests for treatment, or indirectly, as in choices made in elections for policies that will promote their access to health care. It is noteworthy that meeting the reasonable expectations of patients has become an important facet of evaluating the quality of health care. One way in which this concern with patients' views has found expression is in emphasis on measuring patients' satisfaction with their care.

Normative or professionally defined need has been the traditional basis of medical activity. However, the development of a number of more psychosocial models of illness (see Chapter 9) has meant that some of the consensus about what constituted patients' needs has been undermined. Medicine must now debate the relative importance of different patient needs. For example, is attending to the 'physical' needs of the patient enough? If not, how far should medicine get involved with – intrude into, even – people's psychosocial worlds?

Finally, comparative need has been used increasingly in allocating health resources equitably (see Chapter 12). Ensuring that populations are given equivalent resources, say in terms of numbers of hospitals, nurses and doctors, is a form of comparative need. It is not a question of defining how many resources a population might really need, but of ensuring the just distribution of the resources that do exist.

IS THE ALLOCATION OF HEALTH CARE FAIR?

Not everyone would agree that the fairness of health care allocation should be a criterion for judging health care. Nevertheless, particularly for those countries in which health care is viewed as a right and not as a tradeable commodity, the idea of social justice is very important. If all citizens have an equal entitlement to health care, this provides a criterion by which a health service can be evaluated.

Insofar as the British National Health Service (NHS) is concerned, the issue of fairness has been hotly debated, especially with regard to equality of access. There tends to be an assumption that once patients reach the doctor, their problem will be dealt with on a clinical basis, and no fear or favour will be shown to particular patients on account of their background or status. However, there may have been inequality in getting access to health care in the first place. Three forms of inequality have been identified.

GEOGRAPHICAL INEQUALITIES

The NHS came into being in 1948 by simply taking over all existing hospital provision. This meant that any disparities in the distribution of that provision continued. For example, for historical reasons, London had more hospitals in 1948 compared with any other part of the country. The NHS took over these hospitals and, in succeeding years, by increasing the provision of services to all hospitals in a similar way, continued the imbalance.

In the mid-1970s, the government resolved to examine this geographical inequality, as it seemed that patients in some parts of the country had greater access to health services than those in other parts. To remedy this imbalance, resources were distributed to each geographical region of the NHS on the basis of its population size and its mortality experience (the latter as a proxy-measure of morbidity).

Even in countries that have not traditionally placed an emphasis on distributive justice, there are now moves to ensure equivalence of health care access for at least some health problems. For example, in the USA, a history of indifference to equity has meant that there are some parts of the country where it is almost impossible to find a doctor, and other parts in which there are too many.

SOCIAL-CLASS INEQUALITIES

The poorer health of working-class people has already been described (see Chapter 7). Relative to this excess of health problems, it might be expected that working-class people would consult with health services more frequently than middle-class people. However, there is evidence to suggest that, in fact, they consult less relative to their need.

In 1971, Tudor Hart proposed the existence of an 'Inverse Care Law', by which those with the greatest health need have the poorest services. The argument as originally advanced used social-class differences as its basis, though it has since enjoyed wide currency and is often applied to other seemingly disadvantaged groups such as the elderly and the chronically ill. The original argument can be broken down into three claims.

1 Working-class people have a greater health need than middle-class people. Evidence for the first statement arises from measuring various dimensions of need. Although there might be debate about the causes of illness in the different social classes, there is no doubt that major differences in mortality and morbidity (using various measures) are consistently found between the social classes. The same goes for many other social groups.

2 Working-class people have fewer health resources available to them. Finding evidence to support the second statement is more difficult. In his original argument, Tudor Hart used the fact that general practitioner (GP) surgeries in working-class districts tended to be older than those in middle-class districts – which, though it might be significant, was not clear evidence of a difference in the quality of care given – and the fact that as most doctors were recruited predominantly from middle-class families, they would offer a poorer service to working-class people, for whom they would have little understanding. Again, this second charge is not conclusive, although it has some circumstantial evidence to support it in that there are reports of GPs giving longer and more wide-ranging consultations to middle-class and less-deprived patients

(Cartwright and O'Brien 1976; Stirling et al. 2001). Whether GPs recruited from students with working-class backgrounds would respond any differently, however, is open to question.

3 Working-class people consequently under-use the health services relative to their need. There are more statistics available for evaluation of this third statement. It is now well recognized that the working class under-utilize preventive services such as screening, dental care, postnatal examinations, immunization etc. For primary health care, there are also class differences in consultation rates, though these seem to favour the working class (Table 13.2).

However, these figures need to be interpreted in the light of the two other determinants of use: health need and illness behaviour. It might be argued that:

- the figures take no account of relative need,
- many of the working-class consultations are for sickness certificates, which working-class people tend to require more often than middle-class people.

The effect of these two factors is difficult to establish, but relating consultation patterns to measures of morbidity would suggest rough equivalence in consulting rates, and allowing for 'certificate consultations' would support the existence of the Inverse Care Law in primary care (Blaxter 1984).

The problem with evidence that supports the existence of under-utilization relative to health need is that it is not necessarily due to non-availability of facilities (i.e. assumption 2 is not necessary for 1 and 3 to be correct). The argument of the Inverse Care Law is that under-utilization, given a certain level of need, is a reflection of the poor availability of health care resources, whereas, as was argued earlier, it could just as much be a product of different patterns of illness behaviour in working-class groups reducing their demand for those services.

Even if, say, preventive services are offered and made available to a working-class population, they may not use them. The counter-argument is that the offer and availability of these under-used services are in such a middle-class form that there is no congruence with working-class values. Thus availability in the form of opening the clinic doors and saying 'Come and use it when you need to' reflects

Table 13.2 Percentage of people consulting with GP in last 2 weeks by social class

		Males	Females
Social class	I	9	14
	II	12	17
	IIIn	12	18
	IIIm	13	19
	IV	13	20
	V	16	18

After OPCS (1994).

more middle-class values towards health than working-class values. It may be necessary to try other means to influence working-class behaviour.

MEDICAL SPECIALTY INEQUALITIES

Notwithstanding the difficulties in deciding the applicability of the Inverse Care Law to social class and health, the evidence for other areas is more clear. The above discussion has concentrated on social class partly because it was the basis of the original law and partly because it illustrates many of the problems of evaluating and analysing health care statistics. Yet, as far as the so-called 'Cinderella' areas of medicine are concerned, particularly mental and physical handicap, care of the elderly and parts of psychiatry, the relative lack of resources suggests a distortion of priorities in the provision of care.

IS HEALTH CARE IATROGENIC?

A patient goes to the doctor with recurrent tension headaches; the doctor prescribes a 6-month course of morphine. The therapy is effective because the patient gets better, but he becomes addicted to morphine. The patient benefited from the therapy in one way, but the cost was overwhelming in another. The cost of health care to this patient is iatrogenic – that is, doctor-induced – disease.

Illich (1974 and 1978) has argued that the iatrogenic effects of modern health care are considerably greater than people had realized. He divided his argument into two parts.

CLINICAL IATROGENESIS

He argued that clinical iatrogenesis (i.e. doctor-induced disease) is increasing. Thus, in using medical services for a relatively minor health problem, the patient runs the risk of being subjected to investigations and treatments that produce a health problem that is worse than the original one.

This argument is not new, and clinicians have been aware of it for many years. Knowledge is accumulating of the dangers of many drug combinations and of the side-effects of treatments and investigations, so that it seems reasonable to hope that such forms of iatrogenic disease are kept to a minimum. Even so, it has been estimated that 10–15 per cent of hospital admissions in the USA are due to iatrogenic disease, and in Britain a study found that one in ten hospital patients had suffered a medical 'accident' due to error (Vincent et al. 2001).

Some increase in iatrogenic disease may, paradoxically, represent therapeutic advances that enable some patients to live either longer or more satisfying lives despite having a serious disease. In the end, they suffer from the drug therapy rather than the disease that has been kept at bay, and they become a case of iatrogenic disease. For example, steroid therapy in young people may hold off debilitating illnesses, though in later life the side-effects of the treatment may begin to pose greater problems.

SOCIAL, CULTURAL AND STRUCTURAL IATROGENESIS

The second and much more striking of Illich's arguments concerns the wider iatrogenic effects of medicine. These, he claimed, have developed to such an extent that: 'The medical establishment has become a major threat to health'.

Illich argued that the general availability of health care for the population has resulted in increasing dependence on doctors. Whereas in the past people had to cope with their own problems and minor symptoms, today they can go to the doctor to talk, to get advice, to obtain drugs etc. However, this provision of more health services to meet apparent need is both counter-productive and harmful. Increasing the quantity of health services creates more need (by reducing people's tolerance thresholds) and encourages greater use, which in turn is met by increasing resources, and so on. In effect, a vicious circle of need generating demand and requiring yet more resources – which engenders more need – is created.

Some support for this argument can be found in the apparent exponential growth in health services in the Western world over the last few decades while subjective feelings of being healthy, such as can be measured by self-assessment of health status or sickness absence rates, seem to deteriorate – the so-called paradox of health (Barsky 1988; see Chapter 3). It has also been argued that simply making services available encourages increased use. Thus, for example, the different rates of surgical operations found in the USA and the UK seem to bear a closer relationship to the relative numbers of surgeons in these two countries than to any more direct indicators of need for surgery. It has also been found that when GPs attempt to reduce the pressure for appointments for a consultation by taking on another partner or extending the length of their clinics, the consultation rate in the practice tends to rise and consultations tend to take longer. In short, increased resources allocated to health care often only seem to uncover further demand.

This analysis stands in opposition to the Inverse Care Law discussed above. The claim in the latter is that non-availability of health services is detrimental to the health of sections of the population, whereas for Illich it is the converse: that too great an availability of health services is damaging people's health. Liberal health service provision actually encourages people to use the health service more than they really 'need'. Over time, they gradually become dependent on this overuse, feeling it is a necessary part of being healthy. But, claims Illich, this dependence is itself a form of sickness that undermines the good health of autonomous human beings.

The net effect of modern medicine is that people feel themselves to be less healthy than before. The techniques by which medicine achieves this goal are twofold.

1 *Providing unrealistic health goals.* Medicine persuades the population to aim for standards of health that are quite unrealistic. For example, the World Health Organization definition of health is that it is 'a state of complete physical, mental and social well-being'. By this definition, very few people can be healthy most of the time, but many people might be persuaded that they could be healthier than they are. Because an important part of a feeling of well-being

is the size of the gap between how healthy people think they *are* and how healthy they think they *should* be, then a widening of that gap will produce feelings of ill-health.

2 *Persuading people that good health equates to high health care consumption.* The second strategy is to persuade governments and patients that health is something to do with consuming health care. For a government to improve the health of the nation, it must invest even more money and persuade people that to be healthier they must become even greater consumers of health care. Medicine seems to have been very successful in this strategy in that most Western governments have devoted an increasing proportion of Gross National Product (GNP) to health care. Even so, costs and demands on the system are still rising inexorably. In Illich's terms, they are rising because the extra amounts spent on the health care system are themselves generating further demand.

The goal of improving one's health status, medicine pleads, can be achieved by consuming all sorts of health services, including drugs. For example, high consumption of minor analgesics and mood-altering drugs is presumably meant to benefit the patient's health, but it is only recently that some of the side-effects and long-term addictive properties of these drugs have been established. Yet for many years, and still today, patients have been persuaded to take more medication, more investigative tests, more screening, more surgery etc. in a vain attempt to make them feel healthier. In Illich's terms, the only outcome has been further iatrogenic disease and dependence on doctors.

Not only has medicine seemed content to persuade ill people to consume health services, but also, in its attempts to extend illness prevention and health promotion in the last few decades, it has tried to persuade everyone that, even if they feel healthy, they are still 'at risk'. Thus the healthy population can be persuaded to consume health education and health promotion messages together with screening for various illnesses. In the USA, annual check-ups are extremely popular, despite the lack of evidence as to their overall value. Does any of this improve health? Illich would argue that even if there were some benefits, these are massively outweighed by the negative consequences of medicalizing people's lives. Illness and pain are part of the human condition, and empty promises of relief, and inducements to consume, only exacerbate the situation.

In many Western countries, health care expenditure is fast approaching 15 per cent of GNP. This means that people in the workforce in those countries spend perhaps 5 or 6 weeks in every year of their working lives creating the resources that they will then consume to make them healthy. But is this the best way to become healthy? With further increases in health care costs, will the proportion of people's lives spent creating resources that can then be consumed to make them feel healthy keep on rising?

A heroin addict may feel good after taking some of the drug, but he or she is not judged to be healthy. In the same way, patients who consume health services may obtain temporary relief, but, according to Illich, they then develop long-term problems. In the same way that the hard drug problem is tackled by trying to stop the drug pushers rather than by punishing the victims, so, for Illich, the only way of preventing these damaging effects of health care is the destruction of the medical establishment – doctors, the pharmaceutical industry, health insurance companies, hospitals etc. – that is promoting these effects.

Illich's arguments have a simple appeal. Whereas evidence about increases in health service provision and consumption has always been praised as signs of improving health standards, Illich turns the tables and points to their negative implications. In practice, Illich would seem to want the population to return to some idyllic state of total self-sufficiency, but this is clearly impracticable in modern society, even if it were desirable. Nevertheless, Illich's arguments have resonances in political movements over the last decades that stress individual responsibility and autonomy and the deleterious effect of various forms of welfare provision on those same aspects of individuality. Moreover, it is a useful tool by which to analyse health service provision: for example, rather than asking whether a particular screening programme identifies pathology, or saves lives, it helps focus on the possible negative effects of medical intervention. Does screening have iatrogenic effects, even for those people shown to be 'healthy'? Does attendance at a screening programme in some way undermine the autonomy and independence of individual patients? If Illich's critique has taught anything, it is that health services can be damaging as well as helpful, and that in future it is important to be aware of these possible negative effects.

Chapter 14

THE SOCIAL ROLE OF MEDICINE

In previous chapters the contributions that sociology can make to medical practice have been described; this knowledge of the importance of social factors in health and disease can be a valuable addition to knowledge of the more traditional biological factors. There is, however, another strand of sociological analysis that challenges the apparently clear distinction between social and biological factors. Put simply, the basis of this other sociological approach is that because all knowledge of the natural world (physics, chemistry, biology etc.) emerges from within a certain social context, then, to a greater or lesser extent, that knowledge will be marked by the particular form of the society in which it arose. A good example is the argument that Darwin's theory of evolution – which involved seeing a natural world dominated by competing species – could not have arisen outside of a class-ridden, capitalist Victorian society. Indeed, further evidence for the importance of the social milieu to the emergence of ideas is afforded by the fact that Wallace, quite independently, was only a few weeks behind Darwin in devising a theory of evolution.

By examining the nature of disease and the role of the doctor as social phenomena, this final chapter applies this sociological approach (often dubbed the social construction of reality) to medicine (Berger and Luckmann 1967).

DEFINING DISEASE

In any discussion of what constitutes good health, the concept of disease has an important part to play. However, knowledge of the nature and characteristics of disease is peculiar to the medical profession and is usually couched in biological terms. Patients claim to be ill, doctors decide whether they have a disease or not. Yet although doctors rarely have any problem in describing the characteristics of specific diseases, there does seem to be some difficulty in defining what 'disease' as a general concept actually is.

One approach is to break the term 'disease' down into its historical constituent parts, dis-ease. Dis-ease, however, places the definition of disease firmly with the patient and becomes synonymous with the lay concept of illness. This is unsatisfactory, as it ignores three factors:

1 the claim of the medical profession to an exclusive skill in identifying disease quite independently of whether the patient feels ill or not;
2 the 'objective' status usually afforded disease, as against the more subjective experience of the patient;
3 the existence of pre-symptomatic diseases that do not immediately cause dis-ease.

Another approach is to view disease as a 'real' biological phenomenon; this is the traditional medical view. The problem with this approach is threefold:

1 though the characteristics of specific diseases have been identified, as has been pointed out, there is no such agreement on what disease, as a group noun, actually is;
2 great numbers of 'conditions' for which there is no known biological basis, e.g. most psychiatric diseases, are not encompassed within the definition;
3 the non-disease state, by these criteria, is also a biological phenomenon: how is pathology to be separated from physiology?

Although most diseases undoubtedly can be expressed in biological terms, these are not sufficient to explain the nature of disease per se. An alternative approach to the problem is to start from the idea of what is normal, as its definition plays such a crucial role in identifying health and disease.

NORMALITY IN MEDICINE

Put simply, medicine divides bodily functions and processes into two types, physiological and pathological – vision is physiological, blindness is pathological; the growth of epidermal cells is physiological, the growth of cancer cells is pathological – one is normal whereas the other is abnormal. But how is it that medicine knows whether a cell on a microscope slide is normal or abnormal? How does medicine know – with such authority – what is normal? The problem is that the word normal has two meanings.

STATISTICAL

In this sense normal is the 'usual'. It may be given by the average or it may be described by some measure of central tendency.

Does medicine simply rely on numerical occurrences for its definition of normal? It might at first seem so, but there are three difficulties.

1 Statistics can provide no hard and fast boundary between normal and abnormal. They can tell which measurement is more or less normal but not the point at which it becomes 'abnormal'. This problem may not arise in conditions in which the difference between normal and abnormal is clearly distinct, but most physiological and biochemical parameters are continuously distributed and the exact cut-off point where normal variation becomes pathology is difficult to establish, e.g. diabetes, hypertension etc.

2 There are so-called pathological phenomena or processes that are statistically normal in some populations. For example, in Western countries, it is actually abnormal to have atheroma-free arteries, though such a condition is viewed as healthier than the presence of atheroma.

3 There are many 'abnormal' or 'unusual' biological states and processes in which it would seem absurd to suggest that the patient was diseased. An unusual eye colour, high IQ, long hair etc. might all be (biologically) abnormal but still be construed as 'normal variations' rather than diseases.

Thus, the statistical notion of the normal cannot of itself determine which biological parameters are to be considered as potential bases of disease.

SOCIAL OR IDEAL

In this sense the normal is that which prevalent social values hold to be acceptable or desirable. This social definition of normality has various advantages over the purely statistical.

The socially acceptable or desirable is very often equivalent to the statistically common. Thus the concept embraces many of those diseases that apparently exist because of their unusualness in the sense of being statistically abnormal. Moreover, because the socially acceptable may vary for different communities, this definition will accommodate variation in the ascription of disease across social groups. For example, the slowing in psychomotor performance with old age, though a decline from the pattern of youth, is still normal in view of social expectations.

If normality is defined by reference to what is socially acceptable, disease becomes a phenomenon that leads to (or may lead to) undesirable social consequences. (The fact that patients are not held to be responsible for their diseases tends to separate disease off from other states, such as crime, that lead to consequences that are similarly socially undesirable.) For many years, congenital hyperbilirubinaemia (Gilbert's disease) was viewed as a disease – and was treated – until it was noticed that it had no deleterious effects. It was then renamed as a normal variation. In this way, reference to social disadvantage fixes the boundary between normality and abnormality among continuously distributed variables. A blood pressure or a blood sugar level is pathological when it may lead to potentially undesirable consequences for the patient. Difficulty in drawing that boundary reflects the unknown implications of an apparently small rise in blood pressure or blood sugar.

Psychiatric disease, which could not be accounted for by exclusively biological notions of disease, is no longer a problem if a social definition is used. The patient who claims to have two identities contravenes our basic assumptions that people only have one: this break with (our) rationality means the patient is diseased. Or the patient who campaigns against the government in a state in which political dissent and criticism are irrational (in that they contravene the dominant culture) is similarly held to be mentally ill. The question is not whether such people are 'really' diseased or not, but whether the social criteria by which the disease is established are justified.

A social definition clarifies the debate about whether or not certain 'abnormalities' are to be classified as diseases. Is sickle-cell trait a disease? Only in so far as it confers no advantage on patients or their progeny in a non-malarial country. Is homosexuality a disease? It depends on whether the condition is viewed socially as an abnormality or as a normal variation: conflict over its disease status merely reflects the lack of consensus in a society over its social acceptability. Can dyslexia ('word blindness') exist as a disease in a pre-literate society? No, because it confers no social disadvantage.

Use of social criteria to define disease also explains the frequently experienced difficulty of distinguishing between involution and pathology in old age. It is well established that various physiological or involutionary changes occur with age, in particular degeneration of various tissues. Degeneration of tissues, however, is also a characteristic of pathology. In short, disease and involution manifest themselves in similar changes: so how are they to be distinguished?

Whereas biologically these two phenomena are inseparable, they can be socially defined by reference to expectations of old age. Roughly, if the change is expected it is involution, if it is unexpected it is pathology. Of course, our expectations can vary over time and place, but in general our current perceptions of what old age *should* be like – perhaps mobility and a full life or perhaps slowing and withdrawal – will define the limits of the pathology of the aged as against what is to be construed as 'natural' bodily changes. Sedgewick (1973) pointed out that a fungus growing on wheat is a disease of the wheat only because we want to eat the wheat; if we wished to eat the fungus, it would not be a disease.

In summary, although it is obvious that social values inform political beliefs or legal statutes, it is perhaps less apparent that in its very subject matter medicine codifies these same social imperatives. The 'physiological' and the 'pathological' of medicine are only meaningful in a social context that separates the normal from the abnormal. If every time a doctor diagnoses a disease (pathology), a social norm is manipulated, then medicine, as described below, has a very important social role. The fact that, unlike in the law or politics, the codification of social values in medicine remains for the most part concealed has further implications for the authority and social purpose of medicine.

THE BIOLOGICAL BASIS OF DISEASE

The reader who approached this chapter with a firm view of the essentially biological character of disease and the doctor's role may feel somewhat confused: surely, it might be argued, diseases are biological and medicine can be practised without playing with politics? The answer is that this claim is correct but incomplete. Whether or not a particular biological change in the body is socially construed as a disease does not detract from the biological character of the change. For example, during menstruation various biological changes occur in the body, but these are held to be normal. Pneumonia, of course, can kill you, but so can crossing the road or living to a ripe old age. Indeed, it is a matter of (social) judgement whether it is pneumonia that kills or the infecting organism that gained entry to the lungs or the poor nutrition that allows it to be fatal or the cardiac arrest when the heart finally stops. Disease and death are treated as 'facts' by medicine, but they involve social judgement and social labels.

In effect, a disease such as pneumonia can be identified (though not ultimately defined) by the presence of certain biological phenomena, such as raised temperature, distinctive chest sounds, shortness of breath, leucocytosis etc. Diagnosis becomes a process of 'pattern recognition' of the biological correlates of disease; moreover, the biological character of the disease enables treatment to be appropriately directed. A doctor, therefore, need not be aware of the social basis of disease to practise medicine, though this does not mean that medicine is other than a social enterprise.

An analogous situation might be that of architects, who look at buildings through their social eye – what is it used for, what are its aesthetics etc. – but require knowledge of the physical properties of the materials used to construct it. Whether a building is a house, a palace or a cathedral is a social judgement and ultimately cannot be made from the number and quality of materials used to build it. Bricks and mortar only make a building when they are put together with a social purpose. The important point is not that buildings – and, by analogy, diseases – are exclusively either social or physical/biological phenomena, rather they can be described in either way. Sometimes the biological basis of the disease may be of paramount importance, especially when biological/pharmacological treatments are available, but equally it can be useful to view disease as a social phenomenon for the light it can throw on the role of medicine in society.

THE DOCTOR AS AGENT OF SOCIAL CONTROL

Because disease labels encode social evaluations, the encounter between doctor and patient becomes a fundamentally social phenomenon. The patient presents a problem; this represents a personal assessment by the patient that something is or may be 'abnormal'. The doctor then determines whether a disease is present or not. As argued above, each disease label carries a social judgement, so that the diagnostic process involves juxtaposing a social judgement against a personal one. In effect, medicine is performing a social function as well as its more obvious therapeutic one. Specifically, the evaluation of personal deviance in terms of social values means that medicine is intimately involved in maintaining social consensus and coherence. In this role of arbiter of social values, medicine therefore acts as what has been called an institution of social control and the doctor as an agent of social control (Zola 1972). By constantly reaffirming the boundaries of social normality, the doctor serves as a support for the maintenance of social order.

THE PROFESSIONS

A social control function is not unique to medicine: it has been, and still is, carried out by other occupational groups.

The Church

Especially in earlier times, the Church was the ultimate judge in matters of social values and behaviour. The Church legislated on acceptable social conduct and, at the interpersonal level, accepted the penitent's confession of offences against these rules. The confession was an admission of personal deviance that received affirmation and absolution from the priest, who drew from his wider knowledge of what was and what was not admissible thought and behaviour.

The Law

With the decline of religion, the explicit rules governing social conduct have increasingly been taken over by the Law. People are believed to have full responsibility for their actions and, when they transgress the law, they must be judged and punished. As with the Church, the Law constitutes both a body of knowledge (the rules) and a procedure by which people who have broken those rules have their innocence or guilt judged and acted upon. Though the defendant's plea in a court of law forms a part of the assessment of the case, the ultimate judgement of innocence or guilt is independent of the defendant's belief about the rightness of his or her own actions. The judgement is, in effect, a juxtaposition of the defendant's personal behaviour (established by the court) and socially accepted rules of conduct embodied in law.

Medicine

It is fairly obvious that the Law is an institution of social control, but perhaps less clear for Medicine. This is partly because deviance in medicine is usually couched in terms of abnormal biology rather than behaviour, which therefore tends to conceal its social basis. Even so, as has been argued earlier, underlying these biological phenomena are fundamental social values.

Thus, like Law, Medicine is a body of knowledge embodying social values (disease) and incorporates a procedure by which patients are judged ill or well by the doctor. As in Law, this judgement occurs independently of the patient's own beliefs. These beliefs may be of value in reaching a diagnosis, but it is often the case that patients are judged ill even though they believe themselves to be well, e.g. in pre-symptomatic screening tests, or are judged well even though they see themselves as ill. Thus, in the same way that the Church and Law uphold norms of social conduct, Medicine too, as one of the three 'great' professions, can be seen to be upholding social values and, to a certain extent, social behaviour (though the latter is gaining more emphasis).

For example, take the problem arising from a patient requesting that treatment be withheld in a terminal illness. These situations present dilemmas for the doctor because there is a conflict of social values. On the one hand, the general view in our society is that death is an undesirable outcome. (Again, it is worth noting that death is a social event as well as a biological one. In certain situations in various communities – the old in a nomadic tribe, the martyr, the political prisoner who starves himself – death may be seen as a desirable end because it serves to reinforce the integrity or social goals of community.) In Western society, strenuous attempts will often be made to maintain life, though even these may vary from country to country and from culture to culture. In the USA, for example, doctors may stress the maintenance of life at whatever cost more than their colleagues in the Britain.

On the other hand, freedom from pain and suffering and the right of patients as individuals to have some say in their future are, like the undesirability of death, widely held social values. Thus when the patient wants to die, it falls on the doctor to resolve the conflict between the importance of human life and of personal autonomy. In some situations drugs can relieve the pain, and the patient's right to a part in the decision can be reduced if it is believed that, because of the imminence of death, he or she is not 'rational'. (Because the desire to die offends fundamental social values, it is easy to label it as 'irrational'.) The dilemma arises for the doctor when there is a certainty that the patient 'really' does want to die. Then the doctor must act as the arbiter of social values, as an agent of social control.

To argue that medicine is engaged in 'social control' is not to say that doctors are some sort of secret policemen. All it means is that medicine, like many other apparently innocuous social activities such as bringing up children, reading a textbook, going to school, watching television etc., controls aspects of knowledge and ideas that support the existing social order.

THE SICK ROLE

Once it is established that medicine is an institution of social control, many other aspects of the sociology of medicine tend to fall into place. The 'sick role', for example (described in Chapter 2 as a benefit that can be conferred on the patient by the doctor), can now be seen in context (Parsons 1951). The four expectations and obligations really only make sense if viewed in their relationship to medicine's social role.

The patient is temporarily excused normal social roles
The power to legitimate sickness absence is vested in the medical profession and provides an essential element in social control in that commitment to normal responsibilities such as work is a central value of our society.

The patient is not held responsible for his illness
The ascription of responsibility is an important factor in differentiating a medical from a legal problem. Law holds miscreants responsible for their actions, whereas medicine does not. For example, whether murderers are to be viewed as criminals to be punished by prison or patients to be treated in a psychiatric hospital depends on whether or not they were responsible for their actions. Similarly, if a shoplifter can establish that, due to some hormonal imbalance (e.g. during the menopause) she was not responsible for her act of theft, she becomes a medical rather than a legal problem.

In many ways it is somewhat arbitrary whether people are held responsible for their actions or not. Ultimately, it is underpinned by a philosophical debate over freewill and determinism rather than a dispute that can be settled with recourse to 'evidence'. The boundary between medicine and law is, therefore, often blurred and it is open to medicine to invade areas of human conduct traditionally maintained by legal mechanisms. Indeed, it has been claimed that medicine is increasingly intruding into new areas of human conduct and using its powerful social position to legislate on appropriate and inappropriate behaviour. In part this has been the result of medicine taking over the role of other agencies such as the Church and the Law; it is also the result of medicine extending its definition of health problems to include more and more psychological and social aspects (see Chapter 9). This process of 'medicalization', as it is called, has been discussed in Chapter 13 and is further explored below.

Not being held responsible for illness is one of the benefits that medicine can confer on the patient. Unlike many other agencies, there is apparently no need for the patient to feel guilt or failure at having to consult a doctor. This undoubtedly helps explain why many 'problems of living' are brought to the doctor rather than to other professionals (such as social workers, marriage guidance counsellors, housing officers etc.), because the latter may be seen to hold patients, at least in part, responsible for their actions or current situation.

However, as mentioned above, the denial of responsibility is always somewhat arbitrary and it is quite possible to 'blame' patients for having disease. Cigarette smokers who present with lung cancer or coronary heart disease could be held to be partly responsible for their predicament if they knew beforehand of the dangers of smoking yet still continued.

On the other hand, if patients are held responsible for their health, this may encourage them to take preventive action. Prevention, it is argued, now rests with individuals, who must change unhealthy behaviour patterns if they are to avoid ill-health. (The emphasis on personal responsibility for health is also, of course, a political issue, as it makes important assumptions about the control people can exert over their own lives in contemporary society.) There is therefore a stress on personal responsibility in the language of disease prevention. A by-product of the success of this approach, however, might be a decreasing inclination to consult the doctor for these 'preventable' diseases because of the blame and guilt attached to them.

This problem can be seen in those medical problems that already have a measure of responsibility attached to them. These range from people who attempt suicide who, inasmuch as they are directly responsible for their condition, often seem to receive less sympathy from medical staff (though if they are 'really' ill with, say, severe depression, attitudes might change), to the guilt surrounding sexually transmitted diseases for which the patient can be held responsible. In the latter, the feelings of guilt are catered for by anonymity during treatment, while strenuous attempts are made publicly to 'de-stigmatize' the disease so that help will be sought early.

The patient must want to get well/The patient must co-operate with the doctor
Both of these obligations serve to uphold the legitimacy of the social control functions of medicine while at the same time ensuring that they are effective. Just as defendants must recognize the authority of the court (otherwise they are in contempt), so the patient must defer to the authority of the doctor. Failure to do so involves removal of the benefits of the sick role such that the patient is not considered ill so much as a 'malingerer'.

MEDICINE AND SOCIETY

Sociology can contribute to an understanding of medicine in two broad ways. As described in previous chapters sociology can help explore the way in which the social environment impinges on individuals and populations, generating good health or illness. Sociology can also, as described above, explain the place of medicine in society, its role and its effects.

Medicine, however, in its turn, can provide an important window into society. Medicine – its diseases, its practitioners, its organization – reflects the society in which it exists, so that any society in any historical period can be studied through how it approaches health and illness. Medicine reflects what is normal and abnormal, what is acceptable and unacceptable; medicine reflects the wider society in the illnesses it must address and in the forms of inequality with which it must grapple. Medicine also mediates between the broader aspects of society, the 'out there' parts, and the individual person or patient. In this way, medicine enables the ever-changing nature of human identity – biological, psychological, social – to be studied and better understood. The relationship between medicine and sociology is certainly not one way. The future of medicine in its various forms can only be analysed in the context of a society of which it is part and with which it has reciprocal relations.

BIBLIOGRAPHY

Aaron HJ, Schwartz WB. *The painful prescription: rationing hospital care.* Brookings Institution, Washington, DC, 1984.

Abel-Smith B. *Value for money in health services.* Heinemann, London, 1976.

Anderson JAD (ed.). *Self-medication.* MTP Press, Lancaster, 1979.

Anderson M. *Approaches to the history of the Western family: 1500–1914.* Macmillan, London, 1980.

Anderson R. The quality of life of stroke patients and their carers. In: Anderson R, Bury M (eds) *Living with chronic illness: the experience of patients and their families.* Unwin Hyman, London, 1988, pp. 14–42.

Anson O, Anson O, Paran E, Neumann L, Chernichovsky D. Gender differences in health perceptions and their predictors. *Social Science and Medicine* 1993; 36:419–27.

Arber S. Social class, non-employment, and chronic illness: continuing the inequalities in health debate. *British Medical Journal* 1987; 294:1069–73.

Arber S, Arber S, Gilbert GN, Dale Al. Paid employment and women's health: a benefit or a source of role strain? *Sociology of Health and Illness* 1985; 7:375–400.

Arber S, Ginn J. Class and caring: a forgotten dimension. *Sociology* 1992; 26:619–34.

Armstrong D. Madness and coping. *Sociology of Health and Illness* 1979; 2:293–316.

Armstrong D. The patient's view. *Social Science and Medicine* 1984; 8:737–44.

Armstrong D. The rise of surveillance medicine. *Sociology of Health and Illness* 1995; 7:393–404.

Armstrong D. Decline of the hospital: reconstructing institutional dangers. *Sociology of Health and Illness* 1998; 20:445–7.

Balint M. *The doctor, his patient and the illness.* Pitman, London, 1964.

Banks M, Banks MH, Beresford SA, Morrell DC, Waller JJ, Watkins CJ. Factors influencing demand for primary medical care in women aged 20–44. *International Journal of Epidemiology* 1975; 4:189–95.

Banks MH, Jackson PR. Unemployment and risk of minor psychiatric disorder in young people: cross-sectional and longitudinal evidence. *Psychological Medicine* 1982; 12:789–98.

Barker DJP (ed.). *Fetal and infant origins of adult disease.* BMJ, London, 1992.

Barsky AJ. The paradox of health. *New England Journal of Medicine* 1988; 318:414–18.

Bartley M, Plewis I. Does health selective mobility account for socio-economic differences in health? Evidence from England and Wales, 1971 to 1991. *Journal of Health and Social Behavior* 1997; 38:376–86.

Bebbington PE, Marsden L, Brewin CR. The need for psychiatric treatment in the general population: the Camberwell Needs for Care Survey. *Psychological Medicine* 1997; 27:821–34.

Becker HS. *Outsiders: studies in the sociology of deviance.* Free Press, London, 1963.

Beecher HR. *Measurement of subjective responses.* Oxford and New York, Oxford University Press, 1959.

Bentham G. Migration and morbidity: implications for geographical studies of disease. *Social Science and Medicine* 1988; 26:49–54.

Berger P, Luckmann T. *The social construction of reality.* Penguin, London, 1967.

Berkman LF, Syme SL. Social networks, host resistance, and mortality: a nine year follow-up study of Alameda County residents. *American Journal of Epidemiology* 1979; 109:186–204.

Berkman LF, Glass T, Brisette I, Seeman TE. From social integration to health: Durkheim in the new millennium. *Social Science and Medicine* 2000; 51:843–57.

Bickenbach JE, Chatterji S, Badley EM, Ustun TB. Models of disablement, universalism and the international classification of impairments, disabilities and handicaps. *Social Science and Medicine* 1999; 48:1173–87.

Blane D, Smith GD, Bartley M. Social selection – what does it contribute to social-class differences in health? *Sociology of Health and Illness* 1993; 15: 2–15.

Blaxter M. *The meaning of disability.* Heinemann, London, 1976.

Blaxter M. Equity and consultation rates in general practice. *British Medical Journal* 1984; 288:1963–7.

Blaxter M. *Health and lifestyles.* Tavistock/Routledge, London, 1990.

Bloor M, Bloor M, Samphier M, Prior L. Artefact explanations of inequalities in health: an assessment of the evidence. *Sociology of Health and Illness* 1987; 9:231–64.

Blumhagen D. Hyper-tension: a folk illness with a medical name. *Culture Medicine and Psychiatry* 1980; 4:197–227.

Bowling A. *Measuring health: a review of quality of life measurement scales.* Open University Press, Milton Keynes, 1991.

Bowling A. *Measuring disease.* Open University Press, Milton Keynes, 1995.

Bradshaw J. A taxonomy of social need. In McLachlan G (ed.) *Problems and progress in medical care, seventh series.* Oxford University Press, Oxford, 1972, pp. 70–82.

Brimblecombe N, Dorling, D, Shaw M. Migration and geographical inequalities in health in Britain. *Social Science and Medicine* 2000; 50:861–78.

Brown GW, Brown GW, Davidson S et al. Psychiatric disorder in London and North Uist. *Social Science and Medicine* 1977; 11:367–77.

Brown GW, Harris T. *Social origins of depression: a study of psychiatric disorder in women.* Tavistock, London, 1978.

Bury M. Chronic illness as biographical disruption. *Sociology of Health and Illness* 1982; 4:167–82.

Calnan M, Calnan M, Cant S, Gabe J. *Going private.* Open University Press, Buckingham, 1993.

Cartwright A, Anderson R. *General practice revisited.* Tavistock, London, 1981.

Cartwright A. *Life before death.* Routledge Kegan Paul, London, 1973.

Cartwright A, O'Brien M. Social class variations in health care. *The sociology of the NHS, Sociological Review Monograph*, Volume 22, 1976.

Cassel J. The contribution of the social environment to host resistance. *American Journal of Epidemiology* 1976; 104:107–23.

Chandola T. Social class differences in mortality using the new UK National Statistics Socio-Economic Classification. *Social Science and Medicine* 2000; 50:641–9.

Chandola T. Ethnic and class differences in health in relation to British South Asians: using the new National Statistics Socio-Economic Classification. *Social Science and Medicine* 2001; 52:1285–96.

Channer KS, O'Connor S, Britton S, Walbridge D, Rees JR. Psychological factors influence the success of coronary artery surgery. *Journal of the Royal Society of Medicine* 1988; 81:629–32.

Charmaz K. Loss of self: a fundamental form of suffering in the chronically ill. *Sociology of Health and Illness* 1983; 5:168–95.

Clark A, Fallowfield LJ. Quality of life measurements in patients with malignant disease: a review. *Journal of the Royal Society of Medicine* 1986; 79:165–9.

Cochrane A. *Effectiveness and efficiency.* Nuffield, London, 1972.

Conrad P. The meaning of medicalisation: another look at compliance. *Social Science and Medicine* 1985; 20:29–37.

Cornford CS, Cornford HM. 'I'm only here because of my family.' A study of lay referral networks. *British Journal of General Practice* 1999; 49:617–20.

Craig TK, Brown GW. Goal frustrating aspects of life event stress in the aetiology of gastrointestinal disorder. *Journal of Psychosomatic Research* 1984; 28:411–21.

Crawford R. You are dangerous to your health: the ideology and politics of victim-blaming. *International Journal of Health Services* 1977; 7:663–79.

Creed F. Life events and physical illness: a review. *Journal of Psychosomatic Research* 1985; 29:113–24.

Creed FH. Life events and appendicectomy. *Lancet* 1981; i:1381–5.

Crimmins EM, Saito Y. Trends in healthy life expectancy in the United States, 1970–1990: gender, racial and educational differences. *Social Science and Medicine* 2001; 52:1629–42.

Culyer AJ (ed.). *Health indicators.* Martin Robertson, Oxford, 1983.

Davey Smith G. Learning to live with complexity: ethnicity, socio-economic position and health in Britain and the United States. *American Journal of Public Health* 2000; 90:1694–8.

Davison C, Smith GD, Frankel S. Lay epidemiology and the prevention paradox – the implications of coronary candidacy for health-education. *Sociology of Health and Illness* 1991; 13:1–19.

de Bruin AF, de Bruin AF, de Witte LP, Stevens F, Diederiks JP. Sickness impact profile: the state of the art of a generic functional status measure. *Social Science and Medicine* 1992; 35:1003–14.

Department of Health. *Working for patients*. HMSO, London, 1989.

DHSS. *Sharing resources for health in England: report of the Resource Allocation Working Party*. HMSO, London, 1976.

DHSS. *Promoting better health: the government's programme for improving primary health care*. HMSO, London, 1987.

Dohrenwend BS, Dohrenwend BP (eds). *Stressful life events and their context*. Prodist, New York, 1981.

Dong W, Ben-Shlomo Y, Colhoun H, Chaturvedi N. Gender differences in accessing cardiac surgery across England: a cross-sectional analysis of the Health Survey for England. *Social Science and Medicine* 1998; 47:1773–80.

Donovan JL, Blake DR. Patient non-compliance: deviance or reasoned decision-making? *Social Science and Medicine* 1992; 34:507–13.

Dubos R. *Man adapting*. Yale University Press, New Haven, 1980.

Dunnell K, Cartwright A. *Medicine takers, prescribers and hoarders*. Routledge and Kegan Paul, London, 1972.

Durkheim E. *The division of labour in society*. Macmillan, New York, 1933.

Durkheim E. *Suicide: a study in sociology*. Routledge and Kegan Paul, London, 1952.

Egbert LD, GE Battit GE, Welch CE, Bartlett MK. Reduction of postoperative pain by encouragement and instruction of patients. *New England Journal of Medicine* 1964; 170:825–7.

Emslie C, Hunt K, Macintyre S. Problematizing gender, work and health. *Social Science and Medicine* 1999; 48:33–48.

Fallowfield L. *The quality of life: the missing measurement in health care*. Souvenir Press, London, 1990.

Filmer D, Pritchett L. The impact of public spending on health: does money matter? *Social Science and Medicine* 1999; 49:1309–23.

Foucault M. *The birth of the clinic: an archaeology of medical perception*. Tavistock, London, 1973.

Foucault M. *Discipline and punish: the birth of the prison*. Harmondsworth, Penguin, 1977.

Freidson E. *Profession of medicine*. Dodd Mead, New York, 1970.

Fries JF. Aging, natural death, and the compression of morbidity. *New England Journal of Medicine* 1980; 303:130–5.

Fry J. *Present state and future needs in general practice*. MTP Press, Lancaster, 1983.

Glaser WA. The competition vogue and its outcomes. *Lancet* 1993; 341:805–12.

Glendinning C. *The costs of informal care: looking inside the household*. HMSO, London, 1992.

Goffman E. *Asylums: essays on the social situation of mental patients and other inmates*. Penguin, London, 1961.

Goffman E. *Stigma: notes on the management of spoiled identity*. Penguin, London, 1963.

Goode WJ. Encroachment, charlatanism and the emerging professions: psychiatry, sociology and medicine. *American Sociological Review* 1960; 25:902–14.

Graetz B. Health consequences of employment and unemployment: longitudinal evidence for young men and women. *Social Science and Medicine* 1993; 36:715–24.

Graham H. Women's smoking and family health. *Social Science and Health* 1987; 25:47–56.

Hannay DR. *The symptom iceberg: a study of community health*. Routledge Kegan Paul, London, 1979.

Hannay DR. Religion and health. *Social Science and Medicine* 1980; 14:683–5.

Harris AI. *Handicapped and impaired in Great Britain*. HMSO, London, 1971.

Helman C. 'Feed a cold starve a fever' – folk models of infection in an English suburban community and their relation to medical treatment. *Culture Medicine and Psychiatry* 1978; 2:107–37.

Henderson SA. A development in social psychiatry: the systematic study of social bonds. *Journal of Nervous and Mental Diseases* 1980; 168:63–9.

Henry JP, Cassel JC. Psychosocial factors in essential hypertension. *American Journal of Epidemiology* 1969; 90:171–200.

Hickey AM, Bury G, O'Boyle CA, Bradley F, O'Kelly FD, Shannon W. A new short form individual quality of life measure (SEIQoL-DW): application in a cohort of individuals with HIV/AIDS. *British Medical Journal* 1996; 313:29–33.

Higgins PC. *Outsiders in a hearing world: a sociology of deafness*. Sage, London, 1980.

Hollandsworth JG. Evaluating the impact of medical treatment on the quality of life: a 5-year update. *Social Science and Medicine* 1988; 26:425–34.

Holmes TH, Rahe RH. The social readjustment rating scale. *Journal of Psychosocial Research* 1967; 11:213–18.

Honigsbaum F. *The division in British medicine*. Kogan Page, London, 1979.

Hunt S, McEwan P, McKenna S. *Measuring health status*. Croom Helm, London, 1986.

Idler EL, Benyamin Y. Self-rated health and mortality: a review of 27 community studies. *Journal of Health and Social Behavior* 1997; 38:21–37.

Illich I. *Medical nemesis*. Caldar Boyars, London, 1974.

Illich I. *Limits to medicine*. Caldar Boyars, London, 1978.

Ingleby D (ed.). *Critical psychiatry: the politics of mental health*. Penguin, London, 1981.

Jenkins R. Sex differences in minor psychiatric morbidity: a survey of a homogeneous population. *Social Science and Medicine* 1985; 20:887–99.

Jewson NK. Disappearance of the sick-man from medical cosmologies, 1770–1870. *Sociology* 1976; 10:225–44.

Johnson TJ. *Professions and power*. Macmillan, London, 1972.

Jones DA, Vetter NJ. Formal and informal support received by carers of elderly dependants. *British Medical Journal* 1985; 291:643–5.

Jones IG, Cameron D. Social class analysis: an embarrassment to epidemiology. *Community Medicine* 1984; 6:37–46.

Jones K, Fowles AJ. *Ideas on institutions: analysing the literature on long-term care and custody*. Routledge and Kegan Paul, London, 1984.

Joung IMA, Jacobus J, Glerum FWA et al. The contribution of specific causes of death to mortality differences by marital staus in the Netherlands. *European Journal of Public Health* 1996; 6:142–9.

Kagawa-Singer M. Redefining health: living with cancer. *Social Science and Medicine* 1993; 37:295–304.

Kasl FV, Ostfield AN. Psychosocial predictors of mortality among the elderly poor: the role of religion, well-being and social contact. *American Journal of Epidemiology* 1984; 119:410–23.

Katon W, Sullivan M, Walker E. Medical symptoms without identified pathology: relationship to psychiatric disorders, childhood and adult trauma, and personality traits. *Annals of Internal Medicine* 2001; 134:917–25.

Katz S, Ford AB, Moskowitz RW, Thompson HM, Svec KH. The Index of ADL: a standardized measure of biological and psychosocial function. *Journal of the American Medical Association* 1963; 185:914–19.

Kawachi I, Kennedy B, Lochner K, Prothrow-Stith D. Social capital, income inequality and mortality. *American Journal of Public Health* 1997; 87:1491–8.

Kleinman A, Eisenberg L, Good B. Culture, illness, and care: clinical lessons from anthropologic and cross-cultural research. *Annals of Internal Medicine* 1978; 88:251–9.

Komaroff AL. Acute dysuria in women. *New England Journal of Medicine* 1984; 310:368–75.

Koos E. *The health of Regionsville: what the people felt and did about it*. Columbia University Press, New York, 1954.

Kronenfeld JJ. Self-care as panacea for the ills of the health care system: an assessment. *Social Science and Medicine* 1979; 13:263–7.

Kuh DJL, Wadsworth MEJ. Physical health status at 36 years in a British national birth cohort. *Social Science and Medicine* 1993; 37:905–16.

Last JM. The clinical iceberg: completing the clinical picture in general practice. *Lancet* 1963; ii:28–30.

Le Fanu J. *The rise and fall of modern medicine*. Abacus, London, 1999.

Lemert E. *Human deviance, social problems and social control*. Prentice Hall, Hemel Hempstead, 1967.

Lewis J, Meredith B. Daughters caring for mothers: the experience of caring and its implications for professional helpers. *Ageing and Society* 1988; 8:1–21.

Light DW. Comparative institutional response to economic policy managed competition and governmentality. *Social Science and Medicine* 2001; 52:1151–66.

Link BG, Phelan J. Social conditions as fundamental causes of disease. *Journal of Health and Social Behavior* 1995; Extra Issue:80–94.

Linn MW, Linn BS, Stein SR. Beliefs about causes of cancer in cancer patients. *Social Science and Medicine* 1982; 16:835–9.

Littlewood R, Lipsedge M. *Aliens and alienists: ethnic minorities and psychiatry*. Penguin, London, 1981.

Locker D. *Disadvantage and disability*. Tavistock, London, 1983.

Locker D. *Symptoms and illness: the cognitive organisation of disorder*. Tavistock, London, 1981.

Locker D, Dunt D. Theoretical and methodological issues in sociological studies of consumer satisfaction with medical care. *Social Science and Medicine* 1978; 12:283–8.

Macintyre S, Ford G, Hunt K. Do women 'over-report' morbidity? Men's and women's responses to structured prompting on a standard question on long standing illness. *Social Science and Medicine* 1999; 48:89–98.

Mackenbach JP. Income inequality and population health. *British Medical Journal* 2002; 324:1–2.

Marmot MG, Adelstein AM, Bulusu L. Immigrant mortality in England and Wales 1970–78. *OPCS Studies on Medical and Population Subjects No. 47*. HMSO, London, 1984.

Marmot MG, Bosma H, Hemingway H, Brunner E, Stansfield S. Contribution of job control and other risk factors to social variations in coronary heart disease incidence. *Lancet* 1997; 350:235–9.

Marmot MG, Syme SL. Acculturation and coronary heart disease in Japanese Americans. *American Journal of Epidemiology* 1976; 104:225–47.

Marmot MG, Syme SL, Kagan A, Kato H, Cohen JB, Belsky J. Epidemiological studies of coronary heart disease and stroke in Japanese men living in Japan, Hawaii and California. *American Journal of Epidemiology* 1975; 102:514–25.

Mason J, Drummond M, Torrance G. Some guidelines on the use of cost effectiveness league tables. *British Medical Journal* 1993; 306:570–2.

McCulloch A. Social environments and health: cross sectional national survey. *British Medical Journal* 2001; 323:208–9.

McDowell I, Newell C. *Measuring health status: a guide to rating scales and questionnaires*. Oxford University Press, Oxford, 1987.

McKeown T. *The role of medicine*. Blackwell, Oxford, 1979.

Mead N, Bower P. Patient-centredness: a conceptual framework and review of the empirical literature. *Social Science and Medicine* 2000; 51:1087–110.

Mechanic D. The concept of illness behaviour. *Journal of Chronic Diseases* 1962; 15:189–94.

Mechanic D, Volkart EH. Illness behaviour and medical diagnosis. *Journal of Health and Human Behaviour* 1960; 1:86–94.

Melzack R, Wall PD. Pain mechanisms: a new theory. *Science* 1965; 150:971.

Meyer RJ, Haggerty RJ. Streptococcal infection in families: factors altering individual susceptibility. *Pediatrics* 1962; 29:539–49.

Misselbrook D, Armstrong D. Patients' response to risk information about the benefits of treating hypertension. *British Journal of General Practice* 2001; 51:276–9.

Moore J, Phipps K, Marcer D, Lewith G. Why do people seek treatment by alternative medicine? *British Medical Journal* 1985; 290:28–9.

Morgan M. Measuring social inequality: occupational classes and their alternatives. *Community Medicine* 1983; 5:116–24.

Moser KA, Fox AJ, Jones DR, Goldblatt PO. Unemployment and mortality in the OPCS Longitudinal Study. *Lancet* 1984; ii:1324–8.

Moser KA, Goldblatt PO, Fox AJ, Jones DR. Unemployment and mortality: a comparison of the 1971 and 1981 Longitudinal Study Census samples. *British Medical Journal* 1987; 294:86–90.

Murray CJ, Lopez AD. Quantifying disability: data methods and results. *Bulletin of the World Health Organisation* 1994; 72:429–45.

Najman JM, Vance JC, Boyle F, Embleton G, Foster B, Thearle J. The impact of a child death on marital adjustment. *Social Science and Medicine* 1993; 37:1005–10.

Nathanson CA. Sex, illness, and medical care: a review of data, theory and method. *Social Science and Medicine* 1977; 1:13–25.

Nazroo J. Genetic cultural or socio-economic vulnerability? Explaining ethnic inequalities in health. *Sociology of Health and Illness* 1998; 20:710–30.

Nazroo JY, Edwards AC, Brown GW. Gender differences in the prevalence of depression: artefact, alternative disorders, biology or roles? *Sociology of Health and Illness* 1998; 20:312–30.

Oliver M. *Understanding disability*. Palgrave, Basingstoke, 1996.

OPCS. *Social trends*. HMSO, London, 1994.

OPCS. *General Household Survey*. HMSO, London, 1998.

Parsons T. *The social system*. Free Press, New York, 1951.

Patrick DL, Morgan M, Charlton JRH. Psychosocial support and change in the health status of physically disabled people. *Social Science and Medicine* 1986; 22:1347–54.

Pennebaker JW. Accuracy of symptom perception. In Baum A, Taylor SE, Singer J. (eds) *Handbook of psychology and health*, Volume IV. Erlbaum, New Jersey, 1984, pp.189–218.

Pill R, Peters TJ, Robling MR. Factors associated with health behaviour among mothers of lower socio-economic status: a British example. *Social Science and Medicine* 1993; 36:1137–44.

Pill R, Stott NCH. Concepts of illness causation and responsibility: some preliminary data from a sample of working class mothers. *Social Science and Medicine* 1982; 16:315–22.

Platt S, Kreitman N. Unemployment and parasuicide in Edinburgh 1968–82. *British Medical Journal* 1984; 289:1029–32.

Putnam R. *Bowling alone: the collapse and revival of American community*. Simon & Schuster, New York, 2000.

Rawles JMm Haites NE. Patient and general practitioner delays in acute myocardial infarcts. *British Medical Journal* 1988; 296:882–4.

Robinson D, Henry S. *Self-help and health*. Martin Robertson, London, 1977.

Rose G, Marmot M. Social class and CHD. *British Heart Journal* 1981; 45:13–19.

Rosenhan D. On being sane in insane places. *Science* 1973; 179:250–8.

Rosenthal M. *Dealing with medical malpractice: the British and Swedish experience*. Tavistock, London, 1987.

Safilios-Rothschild C. *The sociology and social psychology of disability and rehabilitation*. Random House, New York, 1970.

Safilios-Rothschild C. Disabled persons' self-definitions and their implications for rehabilitation. In Albrecht GL (ed.) *The sociology of physical disability and rehabilitation*. University of Pittsburgh Press, Pittsburgh, 1976, pp. 395–406.

Scambler G. Perceiving and coping with stigmatizing illness. In Fitzpatrick R, Hinton J, Newman S, Scambler G, Thompson J. (eds) *The experience of illness*. Tavistock, London, 1984, pp. 203–26.

Scambler G, Hopkins A. Being epileptic: coming to terms with stigma. *Sociology of Health and Illness* 1986; 8:26–43.

Schoenbach VJ, Kaplan BH, Fredman L, Kleinbaum DG. Social ties and mortality in Evans County, Georgia. *American Journal of Epidemiology* 1986; 123:577–91.

Schur E. *Labelling deviant behaviour*. Harper and Row, London, 1971.

Scott RA. *The making of blind men*. Russell Sage, London, 1969.

Scull AT. *Decarceration*. Prentice Hall, Englewood Cliffs, 1977.

Sedgewick P. Mental illness *is* illness. *Salmagundi* 1973; 20:196–224.

Sen A. Health: perception versus observation. *British Medical Journal* 2002; 324:860–1.

Sharma U. *Complementary medicine today: practitioners and patients*. Routledge, London, 1992.

Smaje C. The ethnic patterning of health: new directions for theory and research. *Sociology of Health and Illness* 1996; 18:139–71.

Sprangers MA, Schwartz CE. Integrating response shift into health-related quality of life resaerch: a theoretical model. *Social Science and Medicine* 1999; 48:1507–15.

Starfield B. *Primary care*. Oxford University Press, New York, 1990.

Stirling, AM, Wilson P, McConnachie A. Deprivation, psychological distress and consultation length in general practice. *British Journal of General Practice* 2001; 51:456–60.

Szasz TS. *The myth of mental illness*. Paladin, St Albans, 1962.

Szasz TS, Hollender MH. A contribution to the philosophy of medicine: the basic models of the doctor patient relationship. *Archives of Internal Medicine* 1956; 97:585–92.

Townsend P, Davidson N. *The Black Report*. Penguin, London, 1982.

Townsend P, Davidson N, Withehead M. *Inequalities in health*. Penguin, London, 1988.

Tuckett D, Boulton M, Olson C, Williams A. *Meetings between experts: an approach to sharing ideas in medical consultations*. Tavistock, London, 1985.

Tudor Hart J. The inverse care law. *Lancet* 1971; i:405–12.

Turner RM. Recurrent abdominal pain in childhood. *Journal of the Royal College of General Practitioners* 1978; 28:729–34.

Van de Meehn HD, Stronks K, Machenbach JP. A lifecourse perspective on socio-economic inequalaities in health. *Sociology of Health and Illness* 1998; 20:754–77.

Verbrugge LM. Gender and health: an update on hypotheses and evidence. *Journal of Health and Social Behaviour* 1985; 26:156–82.

Verbrugge LM. The twain meet: empirical explanations of sex differences in health and mortality. *Journal of Health and Social Behaviour* 1989; 30:282–304.

Vincent C, Neale G, Woloshynowych M. Adverse events in British hospitals: preliminary retrospective record review. *British Medical Journal* 2001; 322:517–19.

Wadsworth M, Montgomery SM, Bartley MJ. The persisting effect of unemployment on health and social well-being in men early in working life. *Social Science and Medicine* 1999; 48:1491–9.

Waldron I. Why do women live longer than men? *Social Science and Medicine* 1976; 10:240–62.

Waldron I. Recent trends in sex mortality ratios for adults in developed countries. *Social Science and Medicine* 1993; 36:451–62.

Ware JE Jr, Brook RH, Rogers WH et al. Comparison of health outcomes at a health maintenance organisation with those of fee-for-service care. *Lancet* 1986; 1:1017–22.

Weiner C. The burden of rheumatoid arthritis: tolerating the uncertainty. *Social Science and Medicine* 1975; 9:97–104.

WHO. *International classification of impairments, disabilities and handicaps.* World Health Organization, Geneva, 1980.

Wilkinson RG. Income distribution and mortality: a 'natural' experiment. *Sociology of Health and Illness* 1990; 12:391–412.

Wilkinson RG. *Unhealthy societies.* Routledge, London, 1996.

Williams A. Economics of coronary artery bypass grafting. *British Medical Journal* 1985; 291:326–9.

Williams G. The genesis of chronic illness: narrative reconstruction. *Sociology of Health and Illness* 1984; 6:175–200.

Williams S, Calnan M. Convergence and divergence: assessing criteria of consumer satisfaction across general practice, dental and hospital settings. *Social Science and Medicine* 1991; 33:707–16.

Wright AF, Perini A. Hidden psychiatric illness: use of the general health questionnaire in general practice. *British Journal of General Practice* 1987; 37:164–7.

Zola IK. Medicine as an institution of social control. *Sociological Review* 1972; 20:487–504.

Zola IK. Pathways to the doctor: from person to patient. *Social Science and Medicine* 1973; 7:677–89.

INDEX